On the Road with Roz

Adventures in Travel and Life

Roz Varon

ISBN: 978-0-692-91235-5

Book interior and cover design by Sarah E. Holroyd
(http://sleepingcatbooks.com)

This book is dedicated with love to my daughter Sara, who has become an incredible travel companion, and a shining example of what it means to be an ambassador, positively representing both Chicago and the USA. She makes me proud every day.

To my husband Glenn, for his support and patience during our adventures while I wrote into the wee morning hours, and took the extra time needed to get "…just one more picture, I promise!"

To Elaine, for her guidance, wisdom and friendship in making this dream a reality.

To all the fans who have followed my journeys—I hope revisiting these memories brings you smiles and inspiration.

Introduction

I have always had a passion for travel. From the time I was a child vacationing with my family at Disneyland—and discovering that there was so much beyond my world in Chicago—I have been drawn to places both exotic and familiar.

This appetite for adventure, and for sharing the experiences with both family and friends has continued throughout my adult life. But recently with a 2006 diagnosis of Stage 4 breast cancer, this craving has taken on special importance.

So many places to see with an unknown amount of time (for anyone), I have accelerated travel plans. Having my family along on these trips has enhanced my enjoyment of exploring landmarks, hidden treasures and new discoveries. Solo travel is not my thing!

It gives me enormous satisfaction to be able to share these episodes through pictures and stories. That was my impetus for writing about each one of the trips described between the covers of this book. So let's begin…

Table of Contents

Travel

Getting Ready for the Inauguration Express 1-15-09

Welcome! Who knew that my first adventure would be the historic trip to Washington D.C. to witness the inauguration of President-Elect Barack Obama? As I wrote this, I had a million things swirling in my head, making sure I was as prepared as I could be for this one-of-a-kind adventure.

I call this an adventure because for one, I had never traveled in a sleeper car on a train. That in itself is pretty darn cool! But the inauguration itself would be the epitome of an adventure. I could plan the method of transportation, I could plan what to wear, and I could plan my day.

What I couldn't know in advance was just how many people would actually be on the mall and how authorities in D.C would handle this crowd. I didn't know who I'd run into, or who I'd meet. I didn't know what events, if any, I'd be able to attend. All of this unknown was a bit scary, but also quite exciting. I was sure there would be hundreds of thousands of people, right there with me, experiencing the same emotions.

That was the beauty of this adventure—I could post pictures and share these experiences with you from the perspective of "Roz the citizen." I had no special credentials, no press pass, nada; just me! Of course, I did have identification and a special "badge" to identify me as a passenger on the Inauguration Train, but other than that, I was on my own.

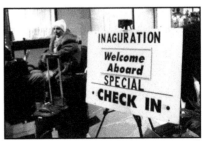

I was traveling with my 13-year-old daughter, Sara. It was interesting to see this piece of history through her eyes.

We're Approaching Cleveland
1-17-09

W e were finally on our way! Saturday night was interesting, to say the least. As we gathered at Union Station waiting to board the Inauguration Express, our group was very excited to be embarking on this unique train trip. We had a very diverse group of folks—some from as far away as San Diego. Many were from the Chicago area and two of our traveling companions you might have recognized from City Council—Alderman Dick Mell and Alderman Gene Schulter!

We certainly had enough time to mingle, as our train was almost 2-1/2 hours late departing. We pulled out of Union Station at 9:20—weather related delays, and boy was I familiar with that.

The crew was most gracious, as well as apologetic, but nobody seemed to mind. We were just enjoying each other's company and sharing our stories as to how we all ended up on this train. My daughter and I had dinner with Alvin and Debra Harvey, the couple I interviewed for my Inauguration story. Talk about 6 degrees of separation! It turned out one of their grandsons was a classmate of Sara's—and they were both in the school musical.

Bedtime was a bit late for me, considering my usual turn down time is 8:00 p.m. We got in our bunk beds closer to 11:00 p.m. And yes the berths in the sleeper cars were tight—manageable and cozy—but tight! I guess that's because my idea of traveling "light" is not what they had in mind in the 1940s and '50s when these cars were designed. Like I said—it was an adventure!

We were in the Cleveland area traveling around 60 mph. We were some three hours behind schedule; partially due to late departure and partially due to weather related slow zones. No matter though—we were staying in the Royal Street Car, which was part sleeper and part lounge, so it gave us time to meet more of our traveling companions, relax and enjoy the snowy scenery. I was told we would hit Pennsylvania in the 9:00 a.m. hour as we continued eastward.

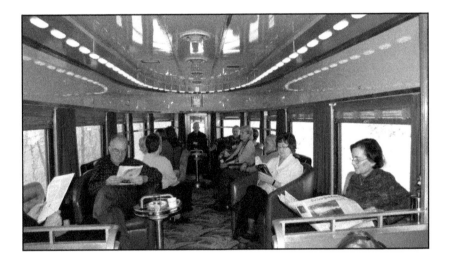

We're in D.C. 1-18-09

We made it to destination D.C. The Inauguration Express pulled into Washington's Union Station at about 5:00 pm Sunday afternoon—about 3-1/2 hours later than scheduled. We were ready to explore! The station was bustling with people from all walks of life—young, old, in jeans, in ball gowns and tuxes and everything in between! Nearly half the station was being closed for private parties.

There were balls, parties and events just about everywhere for the next several days. As Sara and I made our way outside the station, the first thing we saw was the Capitol Building, glowing in the clear night sky, a symbol of what we stand for, making us proud to be one of the millions of citizens who would witness history.

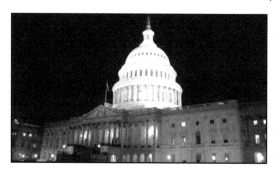

The Capitol was only a few short blocks from where our train/hotel was parked at Union Station. We ventured to the Reflecting Pool, a most beautiful sight at night, living well beyond its name. We spent a good two hours walking around, trying to figure out just where the access points to the mall would be—police and security were already blocking off many of the streets.

The weather was amazing—30s and clear. I had comfy walking shoes, bottled water and a map. Truth be told, Sara really was my navigation savior! As I was trying to make my way in the dark, looking for landmarks I wasn't familiar with, here was my 13-year old, taking charge, saying "Look Mom, just take Louisiana Street to that building

4

with the flag—that's the entrance to the train station!" I may know my way around Chicago in my sleep, but get me outside of Illinois and I get totally turned around!

Sightseeing in D.C.—With a Million BFFs 1-19-09

What a perfect day! Sara and I explored the area all around the Capitol, getting the lay of the land so we could find our bearings during tomorrow's big event. The city was going through a transformation as it prepared to host millions for the swearing in and celebration of our 44th President.

The crowds were definitely growing—that was apparent from the moment I walked through Union Station. As people filled nearly every inch of sidewalk, barricades filled nearly every inch of streets surrounding the mall. Still, nobody could deny the electricity in the air as the inauguration approached!

As we passed by historic buildings, one after another, I couldn't stop taking pictures—and those of you who know me, know that I can snap dozens of pictures of something mundane, so you can imagine how many images I'll have of this trip!

As we made our way down Independence Avenue, we spotted a building that looked like a conservatory—it was the United States Botanic Garden—a great photo-op as well as a chance to warm up! Once we were warm and toasty we continued on our sight-seeing mission. I wanted to see the new "Newseum." It wasn't that far away—my navigator Sara came through again, helping me regain my sense of direction when I got turned around!

This place was so amazing, even Sara wanted to spend the rest of our afternoon there. It had working studios, broadcast news history, interactive exhibits and a rockin' gift shop. I couldn't resist buying a t-shirt that said "News Junkie."

Once we got back to Union Station, the crowds were unbelievable! We were supposed to meet up with friends and go out to dinner, but there was no way we would have been able to get anywhere quickly and we were tired and hungry. Thank goodness the crew on the Inaugural Train/hotel had wonderful snacks on board. It really was enough for dinner, plus it was wonderful sharing tales with our travel companions.

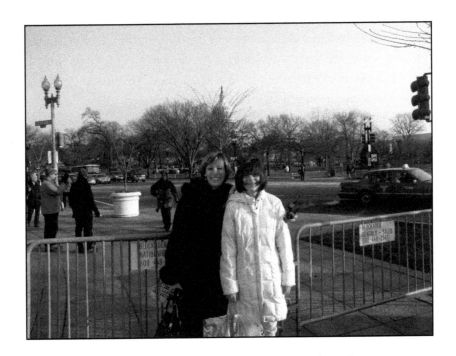

Inauguration Day—History Was Made 1-20-09

I had Stevie Wonder (Songs In The Key Of Life—a classic) in the background. I was inspired, I was motivated and I was very upbeat! Music—as well as our soon to be new President—has a way of doing that to me. I never go on a trip without my iPOD, speakers and extension cords—I know, call me crazy!

Now that I've had a chance to come down from the clouds after the day's events, let me share with you this amazing day. We were up early—5:00 a.m. After a quick breakfast, Sara and I joined the masses, walking to the Mall. We were on a mission. Nothing mattered—the chill in the air, the biting wind, the hours it took to get to the mall—we wanted to experience history being made and witness Obama being sworn in as the 44th President of the United States of America.

I was amazed by the calm, the politeness of the crowd and the helpful attitude of the police and the traffic assistants known as "red caps" who made sure those of us without tickets knew which route to take. It took us about two hours to get to our final destination.

We ended up near the Washington Monument off 14th Street. Still, we had jumbo-trons set up on either side of our viewing spot and we made more friends as we took in the atmosphere of this magical day. When the highly anticipated moment came for Obama to take the oath and give his speech, the crowd swelled with emotion. You could see it in their eyes, their expressions; they knew this man was someone special.

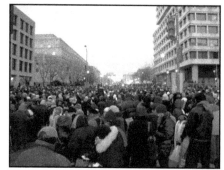

Watching, listening, stepping out of my reporter role, my

eyes became misty. Of course my daughter snapped me right out of that by quickly grabbing me and saying in a horrified voice, "Mom, DON'T CRY!"

A Cinderella Ending to a Perfect Day 1-21-09

After our 10-hour adventure on Inauguration Day, most of it spent either walking or standing out in the cold, I wasn't sure I'd have the energy to attend a ball if we were lucky enough to get tickets. Most of them didn't get started until 10:00 pm. As it turned out, my Girl Scout friend, Susan Rakis, was also the promoter for the group The Buckinghams—and what a coincidence—they were performing at the Illinois Agricultural Ball at the Grand Hyatt. Susan had put our names on the list with "the band!" Whatever works, right? They were on at 10:15 (another late night for me), so Sara and I transformed ourselves and tried to catch a cab to the Hyatt. So not a good idea—very few cabs to be had, and traffic was just gridlocked (shades of my own reporting work going through my head).

Susan was madly texting me, thinking we wouldn't make it. The cab finally pulled up at 10:45 pm—we were in! We took a seat and watched the rest of the set—these guys were pretty amazing. They played all their hits and a string of pop music from the '60s and '70s. After the show, Susan took us back stage to meet the band. The conversation just flowed, and before we knew it, it was almost 1:00 a.m. and we had to get back before we turned into pumpkins.

Now our mission was finding a cab back. After waiting to no avail (what was I thinking?), we decided to take the Metro. Much easier. Who would have thought that at 2:00 a.m. the trains would be SRO with half in formal attire? By the time we got back on our train/hotel at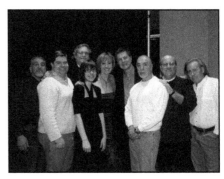

Union Station, it was almost 3:00 a.m. On a normal day, I would be on my way to work at that time—but this was hardly a "normal day."

Our Last Day in D.C. 1-22-09

Doesn't it seem like the minute you get to know your way around a new city, it's time to go home? Now that we'd figured out the transit system in D.C., Sara and I decided to spend our final day doing a little more sightseeing. I let Sara choose. Her pick was the Holocaust Museum—quite an appropriate choice during this historic week. I've always felt the Jewish and African American cultures shared a lot in their quest to overcome persecution and prejudice, and their efforts to gain equality. It was a very difficult exhibit to see, yet something I felt made me stronger for having viewed it.

As the hour approached for us to head back to Chicago, I spent time reflecting on my experience over the past several days. How fortunate was I to be able to take a once-in-a-lifetime trip like this, with my daughter none the less. Even though it was just the two of us, I felt like those closest to me were right by my side. I get my sense of adventure from my father, my sense of practicality from my mom. I get my sense of compassion from my sister, my sense of grounding from my husband. I get my sense of awe from my daughter.

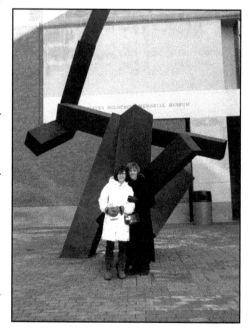

I have been able to meet new friends from all walks of life. Our last evening on the train ride home consisted of lively conversation, initiated by Sara interviewing our aldermen travel companions as she worked on a Girl Scout law badge. The topics quickly turned to our new President and our hope and confidence that in time, President Obama would be able to turn the economy around, fix our broken health care system, improve our education system and reduce global warming. Yes, we had lofty goals for our President, but that's why nearly 2-million people came to our country's capitol.

Life

Oklahoma! The Musical 3-02-09

In a time when budget constraints were forcing many public schools to severely reduce or eliminate their fine arts programs, I felt fortunate that my school district in River Forest continued to offer wonderful extra curricular opportunities to my daughter. Case in point—the middle school production of "Oklahoma!" Let me say right up front, I am not a theatre critic, professional or otherwise—but after seeing the school's production of the Rodgers & Hammerstein musical, I must say "Kudos!" to not only the students, but to the teachers involved in the show.

Understand, my daughter did not have a lead—I would describe it more like an extended chorus role, but being the proud mom that I am (all parents understand this) I went to the show, camera and video in hand. When I found out that the school musical would be "Oklahoma!" my first thoughts were what were they thinking? I'm no expert, but this is a tough show for grades 5 through 8. The vocal demands for the Laurey and Curly roles are challenging enough (think Shirley Jones and Gordon MacRae), but then throw in the southwestern, turn-of-the-century dialect and you've got your hands full.

Well, to my surprise, they pulled it off! This was a tight, middle school production with no major snags. Ado Annie was phenomenal— in voice and comic timing—don't be surprised to see her on the professional stage or screen someday. Every student involved in this production should be proud of their performance.

Being the involved parent that I am, I have ruffled more than a few feathers at our middle school, arguing about policies, excessive homework and the like—all in an effort to make sure my daughter had the best educational experience possible. Don't get me wrong—I do appreciate all the hard work that goes into teaching our children. Being an

15

educator is no easy task, and with that in mind, I would like to thank the entire staff who worked on Oklahoma! for a job well done. Thank you for taking us "on the road" to Oklahoma!

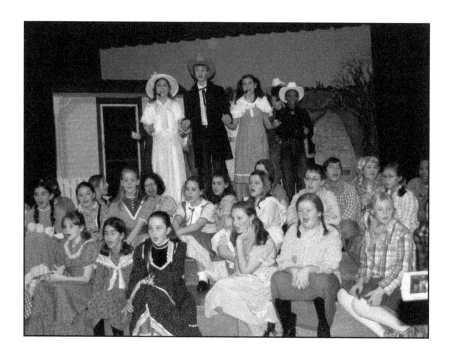

The Teen Years 11-23-09

My daughter recently turned 14. I love her more than the Universe; always have, always will. BUT, I felt like aliens had taken over and I no longer recognized this girl! Let me say first and foremost, she is a good kid; knows right from wrong and doesn't get into trouble. She's a good student, has good friends and is polite—at least in public.

But at home—OMG—she was the evil twin. I don't think I had ever heard the word "NO" spoken quite so much as I had in the past several months. When I tried to reason with her, I got this blank look—like I said, aliens.

Many of my friends who have survived the teen years all echoed the same sentiment—they will come back! My question was—WHEN? We weren't even in high school yet. And then there would be driver's ed, SAT's, boyfriends…IIEEE!

Anybody who knows me, also knows how much I love being a parent and how much I love my daughter. This past weekend my daughter, my husband and I were on the ABC7 float at the Mag Mile Lights Fest. I knew the Plain White T's were going to be on the float in front of us. As we were getting ready for the parade, I grabbed my daughter and went up to the band and asked if we could take a picture with them, and get my daughter's CD autographed (as I conveniently pulled it out of my purse along with a Sharpie!). The beam from that girl's smile lit up the sky!

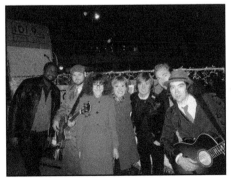

From SAD to Glad 1-13-10

January has to be just about the crummiest month of the year, at least here in the midwest! It's cold, there's very little daylight, it's cold, you're playing catch-up with holiday bills, it's cold, everything takes longer in the winter, and did I mention IT'S COLD!!

All kidding aside, this is the time of year when many people suffer from SAD, Seasonal Affective Disorder, a type of depression that occurs during the winter months, sapping your energy and making you moody. I was looking for a little perk-me-up the other day, so I posed this question to my Facebook Friends: "What do you do to get through the doldrums of January?"

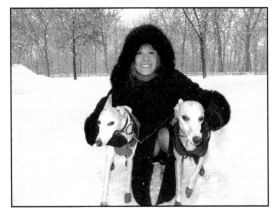

The responses were fast and furious. Can I even tell you how much I appreciated my FB friends! Let me share some of their responses—they ranged from funny and clever to quite practical:

- –Sandy adopted a dog who made her laugh with hugs! (Nothing like that unconditional love!)
- –GrandpanGrandma Micek played "She Wolf" by Shakira and couldn't stop dancing! (I may have trouble getting that image out of my head!)
- –Jane and Jill also recommended dancing (no surprise—they're pros at Arthur Murray!)

-Louise, Sherry and Tracy said working out did it for them. (Pilates anyone?)
-Abby said "Let's move our offices to The Bahamas (Just till Cubbies opening day. Any Sox fans want to chime in?)
-Debra took Vitamin D. Shayna painted. Paula caught up on her reading (The latest Dan Brown book was collecting dust on my nightstand!)
-Tammie suggested roller skating (I'm sure she meant once the snow melted.)
-Tricia, Julie, Mary and Bill screamed V A C A T I O N!
-Cathy said "Spa day and shopping...need a partner?"

R & R 5-22-10

I have always said one of the best things about my job is the fact that I am constantly learning new things, meeting new people and visiting new places. I am putting that to good use right now, by sharing one of those experiences that I had with my Girl Scout Troop.

These four wonderful 8th graders sold enough cookies to pay for an end-of-year weekend trip. Drawing from my travels through my "One Tank Trip" series, I suggested we go to Galena, Illinois. I wanted the girls to experience the history of Grant's home, the beautiful scenery of the rolling hills, the quaint Main Street stores and restaurants and the unique Galena Log Cabins—complete with Alpacas! I wanted to see the wonder and enjoyment through their eyes.

We took a riverboat tour along the Mighty Mississippi. We did some sightseeing and at night some star-gazing. Of course it wouldn't be a Girl Scout outing if we didn't build a campfire and make s'mores!

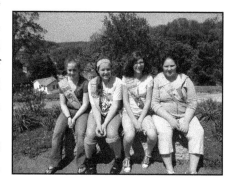

What I came to realize, was this trip was also giving ME a chance to breathe. I had been so consumed by construction stories, special segments and the regular work/family juggling act, I was lucky if I had a spare moment to take a relaxing walk with my dogs.

How did it get so crazy-busy?

I know you can relate to this—we all have our own "deadlines" to make.

I relaxed on this brief getaway. I was up with the sun (which is sleeping in for me!) while everyone else still snoozed. I enjoyed this quiet time—birds chirping, coffee brewing, and a chance to share my thoughts.

A Simpler Time 6-22-10

Be honest—of the thousands of you who lost power in my neighborhood during the last round of intense summer storms, who didn't spend just a little time complaining? "This heat and humidity is unbearable! How am I supposed to do anything in the dark? There's no way I can do my hair without a blow dryer and flat iron! How am I supposed to cook—and even if I could, all the food in the fridge is spoiled!"

And of course, with no electricity, there was no TV! That's where *my* story began.

I live in an area where power outages are the norm, not the exception. After the first one, we bought a generator—not enough to supply power to the entire house, but enough to keep the refrigerator running, and supply juice to one air conditioner window unit and fire up other various and sundry appliances.

The downside to this: my house becomes a web of extension cords, and it's still not enough to power up all the things that make up my daily routine.

The upside to this: it forces me to slow down—w a y d o w n in how I go about life with little or no power. No TV; well, I had a battery-powered radio, an air card for my computer and a smart phone, so I was still connected to the outside world.

But life without TV, 24/7, was a much quieter place. I don't mean that in a bad way—it's what I do for a living! But because TV news is my livelihood, I tend to bring it home with me—ALL THE TIME! No TV means we talk to each other during dinner, not about the news in the background, but about our day. We interact. Amazing.

No TV means I could read a book for wind down time—something I really enjoy, but never seemed to have enough time for, since I'm always catching up on TV shows I record.

No TV means quiet. Away from the noise of the generator, the sounds of a neighborhood without power soften—birds chirping, lots of them—some calls I didn't think I had heard before. Wind rustling through the trees; a calming quiet that seemed to melt away the stress.

And then, as soon as I started adjusting to this simpler way of life, the power came back on—not quietly, but in a most obtrusive way—at midnight—startling everyone awake! In an instant, we were back in hectic mode, resetting clocks, and picking up extension cords. Worst of all was trying to fall back asleep knowing the day was going to start much sooner than it should have.

What I took away from this experience was the need to make a *conscious* effort to SLOW DOWN; then I needed to save money for a more powerful generator!

Travel: A Trip with My Temple

The Jewish Deep South 3-27-11

It almost sounds like a contradiction—Jewish communities in the Deep South. That's what made this trip so appealing to me; I wanted to learn more! So here I was, along with my daughter and more than a dozen members of my synagogue on a "Tour of the Jewish Deep South." It would take us through New Orleans, Natchez, Jackson, Indianola, Greenville, and wrap up in Memphis.

Sara and I came a day early to explore "The Crescent City." We stayed in the French Quarter, which really is a cultural melting pot—French, Spanish, Haitian, African and Caribbean influences everywhere; but Jewish? Hard to find.

Even our hotel, the Bourbon Orleans was the former site of a Convent. We did find a piece of Jewish history during our visit to one of the Louisiana State Museums. "The Presbytere," ironically the former site of a Capuchin Monks' residence, had an exhibit on Hurricane Katrina—"Before (During) After."

This fascinating exhibit documented Katrina through video, stills, eye-witness accounts and items damaged in the flood. That's where we saw a menorah, tallit, shofar and Torah cover that belonged to Congregation Beth Israel, which was destroyed by more than eight feet of water.

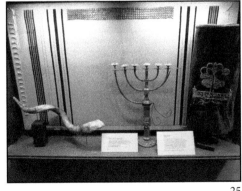

Before our tour with the congregation began I had a chance to show my daughter some of the fun things New Orleans had to offer— the incredibly fabulous jazz music at Preservation Hall, the tasty beignets at Cafe Du Monde, the French Market, the shopping on Royal Street and so many mouth-watering restaurants.

New Orleans 3-29-11

Not surprisingly, the Jewish community in New Orleans was quite small—only 1% of the population, yet it was a tight knit group; warm and welcoming. Our tour guide, local historian Irwin Lachoff, told engaging stories of the 3 synagogues we visited.

Our first stop was Anshe Sfard in the city's Garden District. A Sephardic congregation dating back to 1926 had only 20 members, mostly women, in this lovely, historic synagogue. Cantor Nahun Amosi welcomed our group with open arms—giving us Mardi Gras beads as a parting gift. An interesting blend of cultures!

Our next stop, Touro Synagogue, a congregation founded in 1828 is the sixth oldest in the country. The current structure, built in 1909, is their third sanctuary and many of its elements were original—from the pipe organ to the sconces on the wall.

There were nearly 600 families in the congregation, many of them young—a factor that became predominant after Katrina. Many young Jewish people were drawn to New Orleans after the flood, with the desire to help rebuild and make a difference.

Again, there were many fascinating blends of culture. Touro Synagogue was the only one on the Mardi Gras parade route. There were kippot (head coverings) in Mardi Gras colors of purple, green and gold. In the spring, the congregation holds a very special "Jazz Shabbat" in conjunction with the popular Jazz Fest. The event draws a standing room only crowd of Jews and non-Jews alike.

The joy of Touro Synagogue was followed by the tragedy of Synagogue Beth Israel, the only one that was destroyed beyond repair by Hurricane Katrina. You could still see the water lines, more than 10 feet high on the outer wall. The inside was barren, save for some hanging cables and pipes along with shadows of images on the wall where religious artifacts once hung. A thin strip of stained glass still bordered the skylight, too difficult to remove without destroying it. Even more haunting, the bold star of David, hanging from the ceiling. It could not be removed, as it was part of the building's infrastructure, holding up the roof. Yet from tragedy, this community was brought closer together, as new Torahs had been donated from around the country, new families had joined the congregation and preparations were underway to build a new synagogue.

Our final stop, and by far the most moving, was a special exhibition at the National World War II Museum: "Ours To Fight For—American Jews In The Second World War." The exhibit told the story of World War II from the perspective of Jewish veterans—through personal stories, artifacts and disturbing images of Jewish American soldiers discovering and rescuing Holocaust survivors.

The story I found most touching came from a Jewish vet. Others suggested that he put a "P" or "C" on his dog tag instead of an "H" for Hebrew, because rumor was, Jewish soldiers who were captured were killed immediately. The soldier toiled over this decision, and ultimately kept the "H" on his tag because he couldn't bear the thought of dying and being buried under a cross. Needless to say, a relaxing dinner back in the French Quarter with my Temple family was much in order after such an enlightening, yet emotional day.

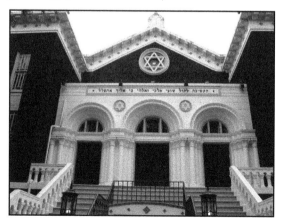

Natchez 3-30-11

Natchez, Mississippi is a quaint town of 16,000 located in the south-western edge of the state along the banks of Mississippi River. The quiet streets were filled with fragrant Magnolias, Dogwoods and Azaleas in full bloom that time of year.

Nestled in between the vibrant flora were magnificent antebellum homes and mansions—straight out of "Gone with the Wind." What a surprise to learn that this city has a deep Jewish history.

Our first stop was Temple B'nai Israel. By the mid-1800's there were enough Jewish families in Natchez to establish a congregation, but they couldn't afford to build a synagogue until after the Civil War in 1872.

The Jewish population flourished in the late 1800's, partially due to Eastern European immigrants. While Jewish residents in Natchez only made up 5% of the community, they operated more than one third of the businesses post-Civil War. Interesting fact—Southern Jews had a dual identity—as Jews and southerners they fought for the Confederacy, but remained true to their Jewish beliefs and traditions.

In 1906, Temple B'nai Israel had a congregation of 500. That number had dwindled to only 19. In an unusual and uplifting twist, our tour guide, Terri Tillman, explained that the community was "determined to keep Judaism alive in Natchez," and they've left a "will" to the Museum of Southern Jewish Experience to "inherit" the synagogue when there are no longer any members in the congregation.

Our tour took us back in time to Longwood. This 30,000-square foot mansion, with six floors and 32 rooms was designed in 1859 for Dr. Haller Nutt, but when the Civil War broke out construction stopped. Only the eight rooms in the basement were completed—the rest were never built. Various families lived at Longwood until 1968; it is now a National Historic Landmark and one of the biggest tourist attractions

29

in Natchez. (Little known fact—in 2010 Longwood was used for exterior shots in the vampire series "True Blood.")

Our final destination took us to Hope Farm, which was actually 2 houses. The first was built in 1775. The Spanish Governor of the Territory bought the home in 1789 and built the addition; but the big story came in 1932, during the depths of the Great Depression.

Katherine and Balfour Miller were owners of Hope Farm at the time, and in an attempt to save the town from economic disaster, Katherine Miller urged the women of Natchez to open their antebellum homes to the public. These tours became such a hit, an annual Pilgrimage was formed and the town's economy improved dramatically.

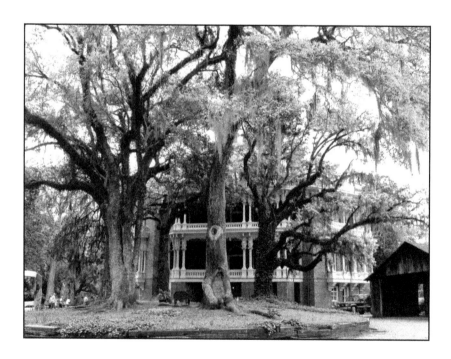

Southern Mississippi 3-31-11

For a region filled with so-called sleepy little towns, our tour went through at rapid-fire pace. On the bus ride to our first destination, historian/tour guide, Stuart Rockoff explained how the Jewish population ended up in our southern states. The first Jews came from England to South Carolina in 1690. A hundred years later they built their first synagogue; by 1820 there were more Jewish families in Charleston than in any other city in the U.S. The reason? Purely economic.

They came to farm communities as peddlers, filling a void in areas where there were no general stores. Once these Jewish settlers saved enough money, they opened their own stores. (Interesting side note: many of these small southern towns bragged when they got their first Jewish-owned store, almost as a status symbol, signifying their town would now be economically vibrant!)

Our first stop on the way to Jackson was Windsor Ruins. Once a successful cotton plantation, Windsor survived the Civil War, only to be lost in an accidental fire in 1890. All that was left was the once beautifully ornate columns and ironwork.

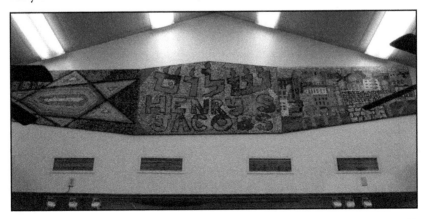

We stopped next in Port Gibson to visit the oldest standing synagogue in Mississippi, Temple Gemiluth Chassed. The original congregation was made up of German-Jewish immigrants. Over the years, as the Jewish community moved out of the town, the number of congregation members dwindled to none by the 1990's. As a result, the city wanted to tear down the building, but it was saved when the non-Jewish Lum family purchased the Temple.

As we wound our way northeast along Highway 18, the scenery was about as rural as it gets; laundry hanging on a clothes line to dry, small simple homes alongside even smaller cemeteries. Deep within the farms and forests, our next stop emerged—Henry S. Jacobs Camp in Utica, Mississippi.

This facility served about 450 Jewish campers in the several states that make up the deep southern region. Camp Director Jonathan Cohen described the lovely artwork and mosaics, all created by the campers. There was a museum within the camp documenting a vanishing culture of Southern Jewish history. The exhibit, "Alsace to America" showcased the Jewish immigration experience to the south. As many synagogues closed in small towns throughout the south, they brought their Torahs to the camp. The camp would then relocate the Torahs to new congregations.

When our tour headed toward Jackson, the focus shifted to civil rights. As we stepped into the former home of Medgar Evers, it was as if we had stepped back in time. The house is now a museum, owned and managed by Tougaloo College. We were privileged to have Curator Minnie White Watson as our host; her engaging stories were filled with the emotion, racial tension and hope for change that were indicative of that difficult era in U.S history.

The house furnishings were historically accurate, from the mattresses on the floor to the street-facing windows positioned higher to protect from gunshot. One of the rooms had been converted into a chronological timeline of Medgar Evers' life, from his birth in 1925 Decatur Mississippi to his assassination in 1963 in the driveway of his home. Evers was shot in the back; the bullet passed through his chest, shattered the living room window, continued through the kitchen wall, and ricocheted off the refrigerator. You could still see the damaged kitchen tile. It was a very moving exhibit, one that I felt fortunate to have experienced.

The producers of the 1996 movie "Ghosts of Mississippi" worked out an arrangement with Tougaloo College; if they'd let the producers use the house for the movie, they would let the college keep all the furnishings, plus $30,000 dollars toward renovation.

The Mississippi Delta 4-1-11

Being from Chicago, we like to think of our city as "The Home of The Blues." The Chicago Blues Festival is said to be the largest free blues fest in the world! We can claim Muddy Waters, Koko Taylor, and Buddy Guy as hometown musicians; but Guy was born in Louisiana, Taylor in Tennessee, and Muddy Waters in the Mississippi Delta, the birthplace of the blues.

Our tour began in Indianola Mississippi at the B.B. King Museum and Delta Interpretive Center. Riley B. King was born September 16, 1925 in a small town near Indianola. He grew up playing guitar and singing in church with the St. Johns Gospel singers. He also played for tips on Saturday nights along Church Street.

To do both was frowned upon, so he left for Memphis and began his career as B.B. King. This state-of-the-art exhibit follows King's journey from the early days. His debut single, "Miss Martha King" was recorded at radio station WDIA, which was managed by an African-American staff.

Being a music lover, I could have stayed there all day learning and listening. I was most moved, though, by an emotional story of this musical icon. B.B. King's guitar was named "Lucille." As the story goes, around 1950 King was performing at a dance in Twist, Arkansas. Things got out of hand and a fight broke out, knocking over a kerosene stove that set the hall on fire. B.B. almost lost his life running back in to save his beloved guitar! When he found out the fight started over a woman named "Lucille," he gave that name to his guitar to remind himself to never do anything that risky again.

Our lunch at the Crown Restaurant was filled with southern hospitality. We were joined by Steve Rosenthal, the newly elected Jewish mayor of Indianola. How did a Jewish man become mayor of a southern town of less than 12,000 residents—70% African American? Mayor Rosenthal's father emigrated from Lithuania. Like so many Jewish immigrants in the south, he became successful in retail.

Steve continued in the family business, catering to all the townsfolk, black and white. When he ran for office in 2010 he became the first mayor to win all 5 wards with 80% of the vote. He attributed this to the good relationship he had forged with the entire community over the years. As mayor, his primary goal was to help residents become more self-sufficient and less government dependent through improvements in education.

We next drove 30 minutes to Greenville to visit the Hebrew Union Temple, once the largest congregation in Mississippi. This reform congregation had dwindled to only 48 members, but they were passionate about preserving their history. President Richard Dattel and Vice President Benjy Nelken told our group how they grew up in an "oasis of tolerance," a liberal community free of anti-Semitism.

They showed us the Century of History Museum within the synagogue, which was filled with photos and artifacts from temple members involved in the Civil War, both World Wars and Vietnam. (Chicago connection: Each year the congregation would host a deli luncheon fundraiser, serving 15-hundred corned beef sandwiches. The corned beef was trucked in from Vienna Beef in Chicago!)

We continued to Cleveland, Mississippi and the classroom of Dr. Luther Brown, Director of The Delta Center for Culture and Learning at Delta State University. Here we learned that the Mississippi Delta region was still a 90% swampy wilderness at the time of the Civil War. By 1900, African Americans owned 2/3 of the farmland in the Delta. Between 1870 and 1930 the Delta region had more lynchings than anywhere else in the south.

We also found out that while the Delta is widely known as The Birthplace of the Blues, it also gave birth to Rock 'n' Roll. (Chicago connection: Dr. Brown is from Elmhurst. He graduated from York High School.)

At our final stop we came full circle. Nearby Dockery Farms was established in 1895 by Will Dockery to produce cotton. As B.B. King stated, "You might say, it all started right here." This plantation community of several thousand workers gave birth to the Blues; their songs would influence popular music all over the world.

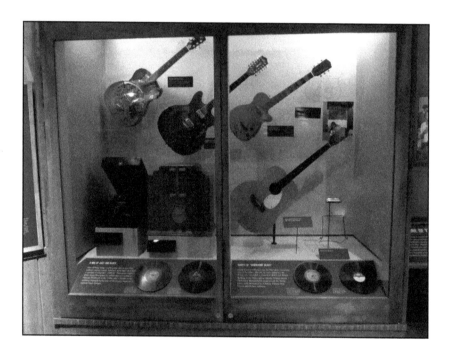

Memphis 4-3-11

The last day of our tour was packed with an emotional wallop. We visited the National Civil Rights Museum at The Lorraine Motel in Memphis. This was the site of the assassination of Dr. Martin Luther King Jr. on April 4, 1968. To say that this exhibition was powerful would be an understatement. Never before had I been moved to tears by a museum exhibit.

No photography is allowed inside the museum; I will do my best to bring these images to life for you. The permanent exhibit chronicles the American civil rights movement over 400 years—from the early slave revolts to the present day recipients of National and International Freedom Awards. There are quotes—from Frederick Douglass in 1852, "If there is no struggle, there is no progress," to President Bill Clinton, "Though we march to the music of our time, our mission is timeless."

We learned how the NAACP was founded in 1910, and how the landmark decision in Brown v. The Board of Education in 1954 ended legalized segregation.

To enhance the experience you could sit on a bus next to Mrs. Rosa Parks and understand more about the Montgomery Bus Boycott of 1955. Or you could sit at a replica of the Woolworth's lunch counter where several African-American college students staged a sit-in protest after being denied service in 1960 in Greensboro, North Carolina.

Especially meaningful for Chicagoans, there is a section on the aftermath of the brutal murder of 14-year-old Emmett Till in 1954. There is also a section on Dr. King's work in Chicago during the mid 1960's, addressing racial problems in the urban north, and the beginnings of the Poor People's Campaign.

Undoubtedly, the most compelling part of the exhibit is about Dr. Martin Luther King Jr., and his powerful "I Have a Dream" speech which had even more meaning in this setting. You feel the emotion from the marches, the protests, and a replica of a jail cell where Dr. King wrote "The Letter from Birmingham Jail" on the only means available—tissue paper.

As we made our way to the end of the exhibit, we found ourselves in a time warp, staring at rooms 306 and 307, just as they were in 1968. Dr. King was standing on the balcony of room 306 when he was assassinated. The building across the street was an old boarding house; it is now an expansion of the museum. Inside you can see the bedroom used by James Earl Ray, and the bathroom where the fatal shot was fired. The bathroom window is left open several inches, just as it was when police found it in April 1968. Chilling.

Several days after Dr. King's death, a wreath was placed on the railing in front of room 306. One has been there ever since.

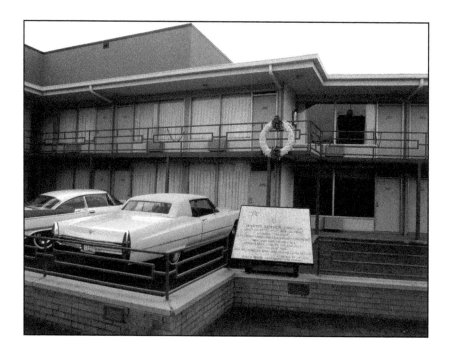

Travel

Our Nation's Capital 7-29-11

This was such a critical time in our nation's history—the unthinkable possibility that our country could go into a government default had a lot of people more than concerned. Call it coincidence, but this just happened to be the the the week I was in Washington D.C. on my family vacation.

Now, I understand this is a news town to begin with—every restaurant, bar, etc. has CNN, C-Span, MSNBC on their HD-TVs—where in Chicago, we're used to sports. But on that week, I'd venture to guess more eyes than usual were glued to those news screens.

I took this opportunity to include a civics lesson in our trip. I had arranged early on to tour the White House, Library of Congress, and the Capitol, which anyone can do through your senator's or representative's office.

I was also able to add "Breakfast with the Constituents" to our agenda—a public forum held by our Senators Richard Durbin and Mark Kirk, where we, the people can ask questions. I prompted my 15-year-old daughter to prepare a question, and was most proud when she came up with one. The day of the forum, she stood up with confidence, identified herself and asked the senators, "Do you think 'No Child Left Behind' is working, and if the debt ceiling issue is not resolved, how will that affect my education?"

Both senators agreed that 'No Child Left Behind' needed a major overhaul. The thing that surprised me, was 30 minutes out of the 45 allowed were spent answering questions about education. Not one question came up about the debt ceiling.

I was also proud of my daughter as we toured the Capitol. We were able to sit in for a brief time at both the House and the Senate. She listened intently as Senator Charles Shumer (D—NY) argued his case regarding the debt crisis. She even asked me a couple of questions to make sure she understood correctly. An educational experience of a lifetime!

Don't get me wrong—we had plenty of time to be tourists. We visited the Newseum (one of my favorites) and several of the Smithsonian Museums from the National Air and Space Museum to the Museum of National History. They were all amazing.

As this vacation came to an end, I returned to work with a renewed sense of patriotism—even though the debt crisis was still unresolved. I gained a better understanding of our government, seeing it up close and personal, and seeing it through the eyes of a teenager. It gave me a glimmer of hope that as our forefathers got it right 235 years ago—our current leaders would too.

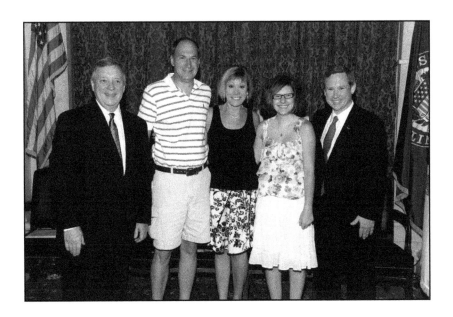

The Happiest Place on Earth
9-10-11

I was on a "Birthday Adventure Weekend" celebrating my daughter's 16th birthday. I took her and her 2 BFFs to Disney World!

Let me preface this by saying I love being a mom—I wouldn't give it up for anything (all you parents out there know what I'm talking about). I called this an adventure, because that's what it was—all the planning in the world couldn't have prepared me for this experience.

I knew it was going to be a good weekend when I realized all the lines at the popular rides averaged 10 minutes! Only 10 minutes for Space Mountain? Unheard of! We hit all the hot spots at the Magic Kingdom, and just as we were leaving the Enchanted Tiki Room to head back to our hotel to get ready for dinner, we got caught in a torrential downpour. It's Florida, it rains, did I bring ponchos, an umbrella, a plastic bag? Of course not!

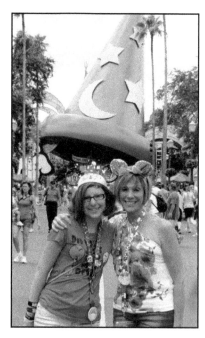

We got to the hotel looking like drowned rats, but lo and behold, Mickey had left a "birthday surprise" in our room. The look on my daughter's face—priceless.

Parenthood is an adventure through every milestone. It isn't always easy, and each phase has its unique struggles. The "terrible twos" are nothing compared to the "terrible teens," But something magical happened on this trip; my daughter, in typical teen fashion, rolled her eyes and raised her voice to me during a minor disagreement—but shortly afterward, she pulled me aside and whispered, "I'm sorry for yelling mom. Thank you so much for doing this trip!"

Later that night, while we were watching the magnificent fireworks at EPCOT, she slipped her hand in mine, leaned her head on my shoulder and thanked me again. "I love you, Mom; I'll remember this trip forever!" So will I Sara. And I love you too, more than you could possibly know.

Life

Breast Cancer Survival 10-2-11

October is always a very challenging month for me. As many of you may already know, I am a Stage 4 breast cancer survivor. I was diagnosed in July of 2006 and have been in remission since January of 2007. I feel blessed to still be cancer-free, and am grateful for all the support I have received and continue to receive along the way.

Things have changed since my initial diagnosis; while treatment is still a big part of my life, breast cancer does not dominate my daily thoughts and activities. I work hard to stay healthy, and do everything in my power to prevent a recurrence, having adopted the attitude that this is a chronic illness, not a fatal one.

I can't say that I'm at the point where a day goes by when I don't think about cancer—I don't know that I will ever be in that place—however, the thoughts become fewer and more distant as time passes.

That is, until October. Everywhere you turn, you see pink—the official color of Breast Cancer Awareness Month. I am ever so grateful for the support, education, health advancements and closer steps to a cure that all of this awareness brings. In reality, it's helping keep me alive.

The challenge for me is, that while all of these organizations are doing double-time to help the cause, it is a constant reminder that I am living with a very aggressive, fatal form of this disease. I think of myself as a strong person—one who has and will continue to be very active in helping other breast cancer patients and survivors. During October, there are times when it is difficult for me to stay strong; sometimes I want to hold my own private pity party. That is so not me!

Breast cancer has touched so many people. If you don't have a friend or family member who is a patient or survivor, I'm sure you know someone who does. What I'm asking you to do during the month of October is be the best friend or relative you can to that person. Don't single them out, instead lift up their spirits. Tell them you love them.

On Sunday morning, October 16th, I co-hosted the ABC7 Making Strides Against Breast Cancer Walk at Montrose Harbor. I was there to support all my "breast cancer sisters, and brothers" at this wonderful event. Let's continue to keep that positive spirit alive during the entire month of October—heck, why not the entire year!

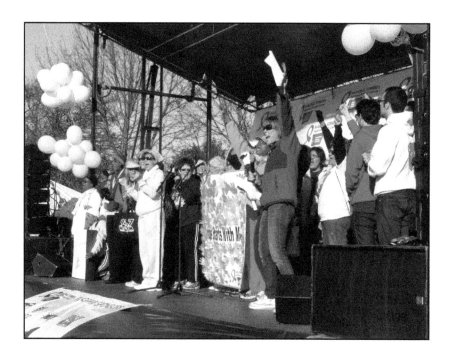

Travel

Israel 12-25-11

Traveling to Israel had been on my bucket list since before I knew what a bucket list was! During the two weeks of winter break, that dream vacation became a reality. I boarded the plane with my daughter and 32 other members of Oak Park Temple B'nai Abraham Zion for the trip of a lifetime. (Our congregation is the second oldest Jewish Reform congregation in the Chicago metro area.)

Like many of you, I have vacationed in several places in the good old U S of A. I have also been fortunate enough to have visited a couple countries outside of the U.S., but never have I traveled to a place so far and so foreign as Israel. I can read Hebrew, but do not know how to speak the language. I have traveled through many airports, but none with the presence of soldiers carrying automatic weapons. I have visited fascinating landmarks, but none that compares with the Western Wall in Jerusalem. I have been swimming in the Atlantic and Pacific Oceans, but did not know what to expect of the Dead Sea.

It's as though I would be taking this trip with a child-like innocence, experiencing so many things for the first time. I wasn't sure what to expect, but I was sure sure it would be amazing!

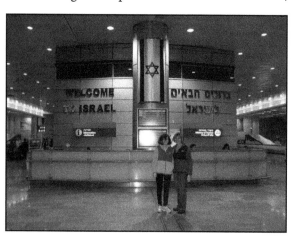

Tel Aviv, Ceasarea, and Kiryat Tivon 12-27-11

This day was a whirlwind of experiences, emotions, and sites so amazing it's almost impossible to put into words. We began in Tel Aviv, at the Israeli Museum at the Yitzhak Rabin Center. The museum is built in a downward spiral, telling two parallel stories—a timeline of Israel's history and a biography of Yitzhak Rabin.

Rabin was known for his peace efforts; the ultimate irony was his assassination on November 4, 1995 at a peace rally. Comparisons were made to the assassination of President Kennedy. It reminded me of the Civil Rights Museum in Memphis. So many lives lost in search of peace and freedom.

We learned much about Yitzhak Rabin—the Prime Minister and Minister of Defense of the State of Israel at the time of his death—including the turmoil in this volatile region and the continuing struggles of so many. From everyone I spoke with before, during and after this tour, the sentiment was that the majority of Israelis favor peaceful resolution to the conflict. My lasting impression comes from a quote at the end of the exhibit by Yehuda Amichai regarding tolerance:

> From the place where we are right
> Flowers will never grow
> In the spring.

Our next stop goes back in history some two thousand years! The ruins at Ceasarea are north of Tel Aviv, along the Israeli Mediterranean coast. We first saw the aqueduct—an ancient engineering marvel.

We continued to the Roman Theatre and the other magnificent structures that once made up this ancient city. Amazing doesn't begin to capture it.

As if that site weren't enough, Bet She'arim National Park, built on the top of a hill, over an underground Jewish cemetery was another marvel. The caves date back nearly 2 centuries, but weren't discovered until 1936—by accident! Once excavated, the public was allowed to explore the winding caves and ancient sarcophagi.

Our final stop was a visit to our sister temple in Kiryat Tivon, one of only a handful of reform congregations in Israel. We lit the last Hanukkah candles together, led by Rabbi Corrie Zeidler of Congregation Ma'alot Tivon. Incredibly moving.

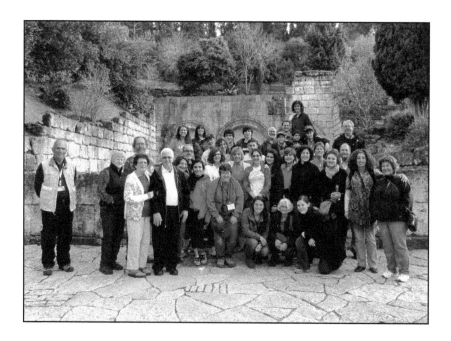

Mystical Safed, Tel Dan Nature Reserve, and Golan Heights Winery 12-28-11

Our adventure began footsteps from our hotel. We spent the night at Kibbutz Ginosar on the shore of the Sea of Galilee. The Yigal Allon Museum on kibbutz property, houses an incredible ancient artifact. The Sea of Galilee Boat, also known as the Jesus Boat, was discovered by two fishermen brothers in 1986 along the shores of the Galilee.

The remains of this ancient fishing boat date back to the 1st century (the time of Jesus Christ) and had been preserved by a thick covering of mud. After a painstaking excavation process, the boat is now on display to the public. It is still being studied for its archaeological, scientific and traditional significance.

As we took the winding roads to the city of Safed, 2,400 feet above sea level, we had an opportunity to see the magnificent countryside of northern Israel, Since the 16th century, Safed has been considered one of Judaism's Four Holy Cities. It was in the mystical city of Safed where Kabbalah, or Jewish Mysticism was born. We gathered in the centuries old Sephardic synagogue and learned that Kabbalah is so much more than a passing celebrity fad. We saw a 400-year-old Torah that is still used today.

We walked the cobblestone streets of the artist colony and ate falafel until it was time to head to our next stop, Tel Dan Nature Reserve.

Driving through the mountains, we were able to see Mt. Hermon, the highest mountain in Israel. At 6,000 feet, its summit has snow year 'round. Tel Dan is a lush, fertile nature reserve, located on the northern tip of Israel in an area referred to as "the meeting point of Israel, Syria and Lebanon." The Spring Dan and River Dan are the main sources of the River Jordan.

Beyond the river are ancient ruins from the second location of the Tribe of Dan, from biblical times. We were told many judges lived within this community and made the judicial system transparent by holding trials at the city gates, out in the open. Gives pause for thought.

As we continued our tour of the northern part of the state, the entire group was thrilled to visit the Golan Heights Winery for a tour and wine tasting. Because of the range of geography and weather in a small area, they are able to grow 22 varieties of grapes, and produce 40 different wines. Most of the wine is sold locally, but 25% is exported. Somehow, it tastes better drinking it right where it is produced!

One more quick stop at the nearby Capernaum Vista Olive Farm and we're headed back to our hotel for dinner and SLEEP!

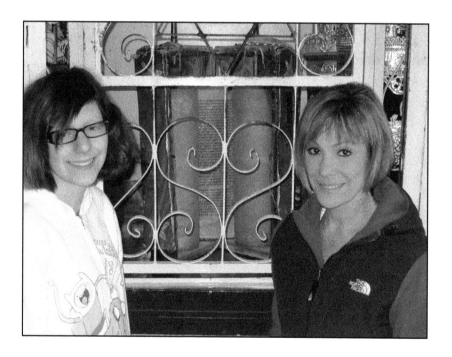

Jerusalem 12-29-11

It is with a sense of awe that I share with you that day's travel adventures. On our way to Jerusalem we stopped at two ancient ruins—the first, the mosaics of Beit Alpha.

On December 30, 1928 members of Kibbutz Beit Alfa discovered a mosaic floor in the nearby fields. Excavations revealed a highly decorated and well-preserved mosaic featuring a zodiac and many human and animal figures.

The ancient Jewish art dates back to the Byzantine period, roughly 500 CE. Debates continue today regarding the Greco-Roman zodiac—a non-Jewish symbol—in the artwork of a synagogue.

We continued on through the Jordan Valley to our next stop, the ruins of Beit She'an. When we entered the ancient Roman city, it left us breathless, each site more magnificent than the last.

The city, known as Scythopolis, flourished during the 2nd and 3rd centuries as the Romans introduced international trade in the region. It was a city of great wealth, but also a culture of great extravagance. The bathhouse, wet sauna and massage room offered many temptations to ancient travelers. From the imported granite pillars to the mosaic floor along the entire main road, the city was one of excess.

When mosaic tile went out of style, the expensive artwork was covered with a new marble road. The Roman Temple was built on the mountain with an incredible panoramic view of the city. Scythopolis came to an abrupt end in 749 CE when an earthquake destroyed the region.

Our final destination that day was the Holy City of Jerusalem. As we drove through the checkpoint, I must say, much to my surprise, this was the first time I saw any military presence since our arrival four days ago. As we approached magnificent Haas Promenade, our tour guide suggested we step off the bus to take in the view. It was nothing like I had ever seen and so much more than I could have imagined. I was filled with emotion as I took in every essence of this spiritual place.

We paused to say a prayer over wine and bread.

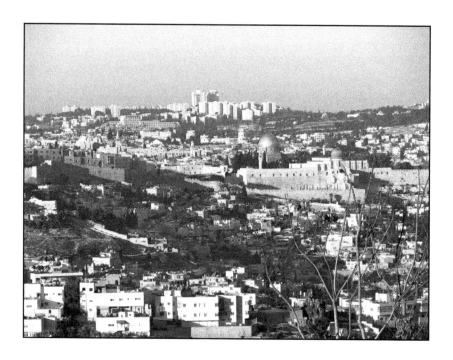

The Holy City 12-30-11

We spent four days in Jerusalem, but I could have used many more to fully experience this historic city. This day's journey took us through the newer part of Jerusalem and several significant museums. We began at the Herzl Museum and learned about the life of Theodor Herzl and the direct impact he had on the establishment of the State of Israel.

Herzl was born in 1860 in Budapest, but spent most of his life in Vienna. An Ashkenazi Jew, he was not very religious as a child. As a young man he had several early careers, from law to journalism. Several anti-Semitic events deeply affected Herzl and inspired him to write in 1896, "The Jewish State."

The book expresses his beliefs that anti-Semitism could not be defeated, only avoided and the best way to do that would be with the establishment of a Jewish state. Herzl did not live to see his dream—he died in 1904, but he set the wheels in motion for the establishment of the State of Israel in 1948. In 1949 his remains were moved from Vienna and reburied on Mount Herzl in Jerusalem.

Yad Vashem is the largest Holocaust history museum in the world. The exhibit is displayed in 10 rooms that tell the stories of Jewish European families before, during and after the atrocities of the Holocaust. Cameras are not allowed inside the museum. There are stories from victims and survivors. There are thousands of personal items, including artwork and letters. I was brought to tears by a survivor recalling how all prisoners at the concentration camps over the age of 10 were forced to work; the Nazis had no use for young children and sadistically made the adults hand over their own children to be put to death, or suffer more killings. I wanted to hold my daughter and never let her go.

The exhibit honors non-Jews who risked their lives to save Jews during the Holocaust. Remember "Schindler's List?" The final exhibit at the Holocaust History Museum is The Hall of Names. It is "a place where the names of Holocaust victims are permanently preserved. The victims, most of whom never received a Jewish burial, commanded us to remember their names. Yad Vashem will continue to collect the names of all the victims, of each man, woman and child, an entire Jewish World that existed and was destroyed."

Our last museum stop was the Israel Museum, where thousands of years of ancient history come alive. When we first walked in, we were amazed by the model of Ancient Jerusalem at the time of the Second Temple. It is an overwhelming exhibit, laying out the ancient city before it was destroyed in 70 CE.

The other stunning exhibit at this museum was the Dead Sea Scrolls. Once again, cameras were not allowed inside, but to know you are looking at pieces of the oldest known biblical manuscripts in existence (150 BCE to 70 CE) is something of a miracle.

On our way back to the hotel, we needed some levity—so, our wonderful tour guide, Arie, stopped at Shuk Mahane Yehuda. This is a very large, open-air market, selling fruit, pastries, cheese, fish, clothing, and much more. The thing was, this day was Friday—Shabbat—and everything shuts down by sundown! These merchants needed to sell everything NOW, and the buyers knew it. Controlled chaos at its best.

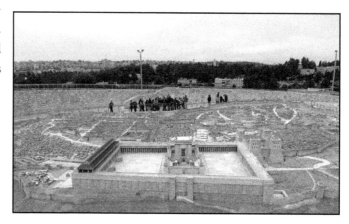

The Old City 12-31-11

What a way to ring in 2012! On the last day of 2011, we had our first walking tour of The Old City, aka, Old Jerusalem. A short walk from our hotel, we passed by some amazing architecture. The YMCA Hotel was designed in Art Deco by Arthur Loomis Harmon, the same architect who designed the Empire State Building. Across the street is the prestigious King David Hotel.

We took a short cut through the very modern Mamilla Mall, and entered The Old City through the Jaffa gate on our way to the Christian Quarter—one of four uneven quarters that make up this city within a city.

Once inside, it was as if we'd entered another world in another time. Street vendors lined narrow roads, ornate arches lead to more shops until we reached our destination.

This was the site where the crucifixion of Jesus is said to have occurred. We saw visitors from all over the world wait in long lines to worship at the Alter of The Crucifixion.

Below us, and just inside the entrance was the Stone of Anointing, which tradition states was the place where the body of Jesus was purified for burial. We were also shown the tomb where it is said Jesus was buried.

Seventeen different denominations share this massive space—some with a room, some with an entire floor. Muslim guards lock the towering wooden doors every night at midnight and reopen them the next morning at 2:00 am. The keys have been in the hands of the same family for 900 years!

We then made our way through the bazaar for some hummus and shopping.

Make that successful shopping!

On the walk back to the hotel, a small group of us couldn't resist a peek inside the King David Hotel, even if the closest we got to "rubbing elbows with royalty" was taking pictures of their signatures. Our New Year's Eve dinner was with a small group at the trendy Ben Yahuda Street. Goodbye 2011!

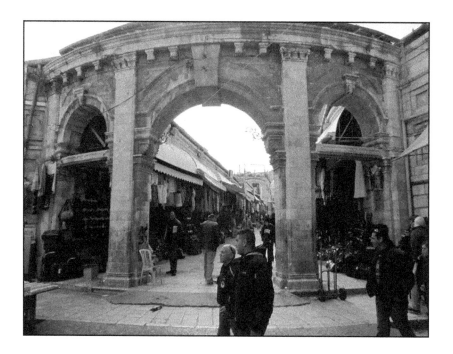

New Year's Day 1-1-12

A clear, blue sky greeted us on this sunny New Year's Day. I had been anticipating this visit to the Western Wall for quite some time, absolutely thrilled to be starting 2012 at such a historic site. I had prepared prayers in my mind, ready to insert my slip of paper into the ancient rocks. I was ready to take notes, ready to take pictures—I was totally unprepared for the emotional reaction I would have, visiting this holy place.

Our bus stopped at an overlook to Mount of Olives, a mountain ridge in The Old City of Jerusalem that is home to the Dome of The Rock. This Golden Dome was built in 691 CE and is said to sit on the site where Abraham prepared to sacrifice his son Isaac. It is known as the site of the Holy of Holies during the Temple Period. The oldest Jewish cemetery in the world is on Mount of Olives, dating back some 3,000 years.

The 2nd Temple was built in in 516 BCE to replace Solomon's Temple after its destruction, and became a massive complex to accommodate the increasing Jewish population wanting to be near the Holy of Holies. The Romans destroyed Jerusalem and its Temple in 70 CE. The lower levels of the Western Wall are part of the few remains from the huge complex.

We started our tour by getting our bearings. Our amazing tour guide Arie gave us a visual of the "before" and "now" of the southeast corner of the complex. The Western Huldah Gate was once a main entrance. Inspired by these events, our group sang a prayer as we climbed the stairs.

Before we went to the Western Wall, we got an amazing view of the tunnels under the wall. We learned that the wall did not start as a religious structure, but actually as a retaining wall for the nearby Muslim neighborhood that was built in ancient times.

As we made our way through the narrow tunnels, we also learned that the length of the 1,860 ft. wall is made up of HUGE 36-foot stones—the cornerstones weighing up to 50-tons! We then came upon something I wasn't expecting—a prayer wall on the other side of the site of the Holy of Holies.

I quickly fumbled for my reporter's notebook and tore out a piece of paper. Not wanting to be disrespectful to the other women praying at the wall, I tried to find the words for a prayer. I was overcome with emotion, yet found a way to put my thoughts on paper and insert them between the stones on the wall.

It took me a moment to recover from this surreal experience. We got to the end of the tunnel, made our way back through the neighborhood above, and prepared for an experience I would remember for the rest of my life.

My daughter and I shared a moment to reflect on what our individual prayers would say. We sat, thoughtfully wrote them down, and made our way to the women's side of the wall. As Sara approached the wall she put one hand, then both hand against the stone. She took her time; I could only imagine what was going through her mind as she carefully placed the piece of paper between the rocks.

As she turned back to approach me, I could see she had been crying. That set my tears in motion as I made my way to the wall. I bowed my head and put my hands against the structure. My mind was racing trying to recite in my head the prayers I had put into words. Tears were streaming down my face. I placed the paper in between the stones and turned around with a sense of calm. It was the most powerful moment in my life. What a way to start the year!

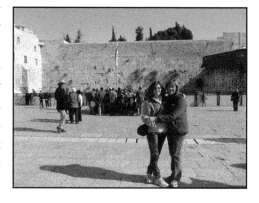

Masada 1-2-12

We bade a fond farewell to Jerusalem as we made our way to the West Bank—destination, Masada. Within miles of leaving the city, the terrain made a drastic change. We passed the Qumran Caves where the Dead Sea Scrolls were found.

Before making our way to Masada, we stopped at Ein Gedi Nature Reserve and National Park. This picturesque oasis within the Judean Desert dates back to the Biblical Era. It is filled with serene waterfalls throughout the rocky hills. As we began our hike, we came across several ibex wild goats looking for a mid-morning snack.

Before it was time to head to historic Mesada, we stopped several times along the way to take in the beauty of each waterfall overlooking the Dead Sea. The ruins at Masada are all that is left from the massive complex that was built by King Herod in 37 BCE.

After his death in the 1st century, a group of Jewish extremists took over Masada during the Jewish-Roman War against the Roman Empire.

The Romans, determined to break through the seemingly unreachable complex, over the course of three years, built a ramp to conquer the fortress. When the Jewish extremists realized they had been defeated, rather than die at the hands of their enemies, we are told the 961 people living there committed suicide.

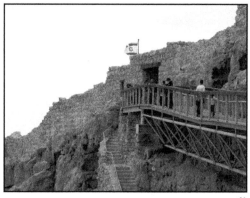

Today, visitors from all over the world hike, or take the cable car up to the top of Masada to walk through the ancient historic site. It is a challenging trail, but incredibly rewarding. In case you were wondering, we took the cable car back down!

The Negev Desert 1-3-12

If you think ocean water is salty, try swimming in the Dead Sea! It was an interesting start to our day. After a quick breakfast, we rushed to the shores of the famed body of water. A little background here—the Dead Sea is 32% minerals, and almost 9 times saltier than ocean water.

Even though it was a little cool for swimming (not to the young people in our group, of course) I had to experience this phenomenon. Adjusting to the cold was challenging, but floating in this salty body of water was so worth it; kind of like swimming through gelatin, but not quite that thick.

Our journey took us deeper into the Negev Desert, and into higher elevations. We stopped at Mount Sodom, a mountain that is made entirely out of rock salt! Not that we didn't believe our tour guide, Arie, but most of us had to do the "tourist thing," and stick our tongues on the rock to be sure. It *was* salty! Did I take a rock with me as a souvenir? You better believe it!

We continued on through the winding roads taking in the majestic scenery until our next stop at the "small crater." While most craters are caused by things like meteorites, volcanic activity, or explosions, there are a very small minority called makhtesh. These craters are created by geological erosion. There are only seven makhtesh in the world—five of them including the "small crater" are found in Israel.

As we got to better understand the physical attributes of Israel, we also learned more of its political history. Our next stop took us to the gravesite of David Ben-Gurion—the man who formally proclaimed the establishment of the State of Israel in May of 1948.

This major event connected the dots from our earlier visit at the Herzl Museum. While Theodor Herzl created the dream of establishing a Jewish State, Ben-Gurion implemented it. The gravesite of Ben-

Gurion and his wife Paula are overlooking the Negev Desert; behind them Ben-Gurion University casts a watchful eye. Before we left, our group placed stones on the graves—a Jewish tradition—and recited the Mourner's Kaddish.

Through the years, Ben-Gurion made many contributions to Israel, including the consolidation of all the state's militias to one national army, the Israel Defense Force. We passed by an IDF facility on our way to Mitzpe Ramon, where we spent the night.

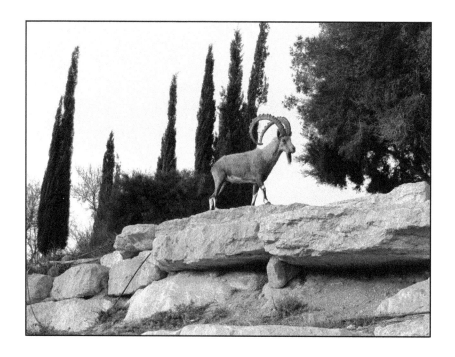

Eilat 1-4-12

I thought this day was going to be an easy-paced one, with a few stops on our way to the town of Eilat, Israel's southern most city, located on the northern tip of the Red Sea. It started out simple enough with a fascinating visit to Kibbutz Lotan, an eco-friendly Kibbutz.

We took a tour of the prototype village with environmentally friendly homes, built to withstand the extreme heat and cold temperatures of the Arava Valley. These buildings use as little as 1/8th the energy of a standard building. The guide showed us solar stoves, an environmental theme park, and an organic herb garden.

We tried our hand at making earth bricks out of dirt, straw, and water—that was a big hit with kids of all ages in our group. After a rich experience at the Kibbutz, Arie, our tour guide, not being one to pass up an opportunity, made a stop along the way for some of the "best ice cream in Israel." We agreed!

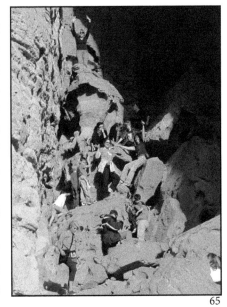

As we continued our trek south, we were in awe of the towering rock formations at Solomon's Pillars in the Timna Valley. Originally an ancient copper mine, these statuesque pillars were created naturally by centuries of water erosion and wind.

Who could resist climbing these ancient rocks? Not us!

After we worked off our lunch, before heading to our hotel, we were ready for one more site—Mt. Yeas. From the top of this mountain you could see four countries—Israel, Jordan, Saudi Arabia and Egypt. Thing is, the bus only got us so far. We had to hike the rest of the way up, and it was pretty steep.

I don't think we were expecting that, and being at the end of the day, it was a bit of a challenge—but we accepted that challenge, and made it to the top! Not only did we have an incredible view, but we witnessed a magnificent sunset on the way back down.

Petra 1-5-12

As I looked out the window from our hotel, the sun glistened over the Red Sea. It was a bright, beautiful morning—a perfect day to tour the ancient city of Petra in Jordan. We had to get an early start, because crossing the border would be quite a process.

We checked in at the main crossing gate and had to hand over our passports while Jordanian officials processed the paperwork that would allow us to visit their country. Although we had been told of this procedure in advance, it was still a bit unnerving to be without a passport. After about an hour of waiting, our passports were returned and we were on the bus, driving through Jordan to the amazing city of Petra.

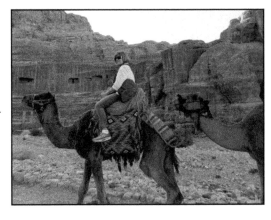

We wound our way up the mountains, taking in the scenery. "Petra" is the Greek word for "rock." The city of Petra is an archeological wonder, with all of the buildings carved right into the rocks. This ancient city is so amazing; it's one of the "New Seven Wonders of the World!"

Once we arrived, it was a short walk to the entrance. There is evidence that this area was inhabited as early as 1600 BCE. At its peak in the 1st century BCE, Petra's population was estimated at 45,000 to 50,000 people.

As we made our way down the narrow "canyon" we were struck by the brilliant colors in the rock formations. Our guide explained that many of these structures were mausoleums. He showed us the original stones alone the path, as well as the extensive water canal system.

When we came to the end of the canyon, the towering rocks appeared to separate, opening up to the magnificent structure known as "The Treasury." If you're thinking you've seen this somewhere before, you probably have. It was used in the film "Indiana Jones and the Last Crusade" as the temple housing the Holy Grail!

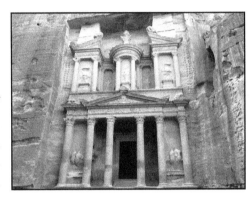

This incredible building, also believed to have been a mausoleum, took 20 years to build with 100 men working on it each day. There are many influences in its style, including Egyptian, Persian, Babylonian, Mesopotamian, and Greek. We continued on to the Necropolis—or "City of the Dead" which displays more mausoleums.

At one point, a member of our group asked, if all these buildings were to house the dead, where did the living reside? We were told, that they actually lived on the hills near Petra, but because these were free-standing homes (not carved in the rock) they were destroyed over time.

The grand Amphitheater was originally constructed in the 1st Century BCE for religious purposes, but when the Romans took over Petra in 106 CE they used it for entertainment.

After learning about the history of the region, we had some free time to explore, including riding a camel! By the time we walked back to the bus, we were pretty tuckered out. We stopped for a fabulous lunch and were treated to another outstanding sunset over the Jordanian mountains. Getting across the border back into Israel was fairly quick, compared to the morning experience.

The Red Sea 1-6-12

We celebrated our last day in Israel with mixed emotions. The members of our congregation had enjoyed each other's company for almost 2 weeks and didn't want this adventure to end. On the other hand, we did miss our homes, our families and for many of us, our pets! We decided to go out with a bang and take a lunch cruise on the Red Sea.

We boarded our ship, the Zorba, at the Eilat Marina a few blocks from our hotel. The ship was built in 1918; today it is used strictly for tourist cruises. We couldn't have had a more perfect day—bright sunshine, warm temperatures and tranquil waters. From our vantage point we could see Egypt, Jordan and of course, Israel.

As we sailed, I began reflecting about our group of 34 and how we had changed over the past 12 days. When we began our trip, we were several families—we were now one. Many of us didn't know each other—we had now learned something about each one of us:

–Sarah loves to salsa—now Jim does too…and Iris, Lisa, Robin and Susan!

–Ben was the most articulate 13 year old I'd ever met—he taught me a thing or two on my Mac!

–Robin did not have a religious upbringing, barely celebrating the Jewish holidays; she went on to become a Rabbi at a large Conservative Congregation in the western suburbs—a true inspiration.

–Caleb celebrated his 18th birthday on our trip—L'Chiam!

–Like many of the teens on our trip, Rachel and Sara saw each other on occasion at school or at the temple; their friendship was now a special one, with many shared memories, from the sea to the sky.

–Cantor Julie had done an amazing job organizing this trip.

This trip made an impact on my life in many ways, from historical to spiritual, but it wouldn't have been the same without this special group of people—my extended temple family. Each of them touched my life, and I thank them for that. I made the journey back home with renewed faith, a fresh outlook and gratitude for my new friends—my new family. Shalom.

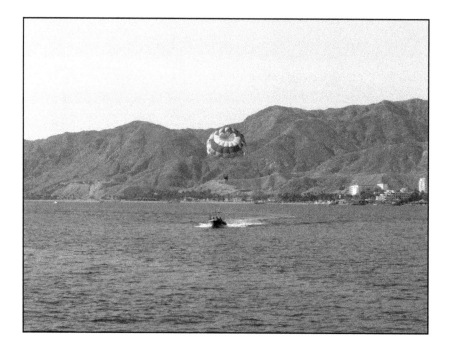

Travel

Ireland 3-25-12

Want to know your teen better? Go on a trip with them! Want some insight into your teen's world? Go on a trip with them, and 40 of their peers as a parent chaperone! My initial intention when I signed on as a chaperone for the Oak Park River Forest High School (OPRFHS) choir students' trip to Ireland was a tad self-serving...a chance to see a magnificent country for the first time, and spend some (very limited) time with my daughter. It had turned into much more.

Our first two days were a whirlwind of history, foliage and fun sprinkled with jet lag. Each chaperone had four students in their group. We began our adventure at The Rock of Cashel in County Tipperary. This historic site was the seat of kings from the 4th century until 1101 when it was presented to the church. Talk about ancient artifact!

At the end of our tour we made our way to Cork for dinner and some well needed sleep.

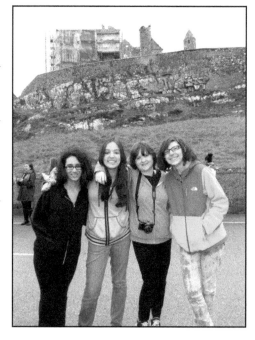

By our second day, many of us were adjusting to the five-hour time difference— good thing, because we were on our way to the Blarney Castle & Gardens to climb the narrow stairs that led to the top of the castle to kiss "the Blarney Stone" (Like I really need any help in the gift of gab department!).

The odd thing is, tradition requires you to lie on your back and bend backwards to "kiss the stone" nearly upside down! I guess, "when in Rome" right? The gardens were absolutely amazing—60 acres of the most brilliant hues you could imagine. The greenery is everything you've heard about and then some. The "Emerald Isle" doesn't begin to cover the richness of the deep green foliage that surrounded us.

Before leaving the area, we shopped 'til we dropped at Blarney Woolen Mills—"The Largest Irish Gift Shop in the World!"

Our day wrapped up at Killarney National Park—an incredible 26,000 acres, filled with mountains, lakes, woodlands and waterfalls. The fresh air was intoxicating. The serene beauty was beyond magnificent.

The Ring of Kerry 3-26-12

The more things change, the more they stay the same. When my generation was 16, we didn't have cell phones, laptops, or any of the other technology that preoccupies today's teens. However—it's been my observation—especially on this trip with 40 teens that the conflicts, struggles and ultimate rewards are pretty much the same. One minute I was having an intellectually compelling conversation with a student, the next, the kids shrieked with delight as our bus passed a flock of sheep grazing on the rocky hillside; and in Ireland, that happens every few minutes!

Day Three took us through the Ring of Kerry, an incredibly scenic circular route; encompassing 180 km of castles, historic homes, and quaint villages nestled within several peninsulas. Our delightful guide, Liam, with his magically lyrical Irish brogue, surprised the students by stopping at a sheep farm for a herding demonstration given by Brendan Ferris and his award winning border collies.

This eventful day culminated with the students performing in their first concert at St. Mary's Church in Killarney; a very moving concert. We, as parents and music lovers, could not have been more proud.

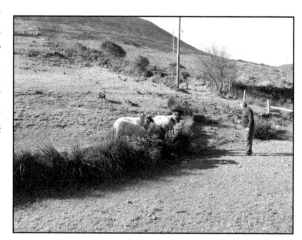

Galway 3-27-12

I don't know which part of this Ireland trip I found more exciting—the adventure seen through my eyes, discovering this lush and magnificent country with a fascinating history? Or, seeing it through my daughter's eyes—a new experience around every turn—from the early morning mist that greeted us each day, to the genuine warmth of the Irish people who were so kind and welcoming to this group of Americans.

As Day Four began, we said goodbye to Killarney and hello to Galway. We got there via ferry on the River Shannon, the largest river in Ireland ("You mean the bus goes on the ferry too?") We made our way to the Cliffs of Moher, a magical vista along the Atlantic Ocean on

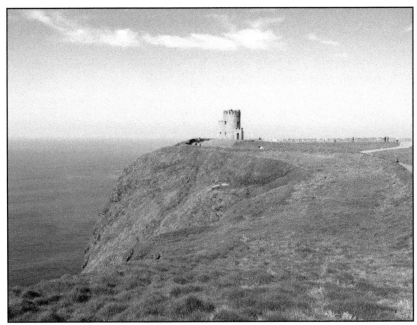

the western seaboard of County Clare, an incredible natural structure that was formed 320 million years ago.

We explored O'Brien's Tower, which was built in 1835 as a viewing point for tourists. On a clear day you can see five counties—but not as far as Boston, as our tour guide jokingly suggested.

We continued on to the amazing Poulnabrone Dolmen. A "dolmen" is an ancient tomb—"Poulnabrone" translates to "hole of sorrows" in Irish. This burial ground dates back to the Neolithic Period, 4200 BC—2900 BC. During the most recent excavation in 1985, 33 bodies were found buried under the monument.

Because of the uneven way sunlight hit the jagged rocks, this is the only place in the world, we were told, where plants from the Mediterranean grow alongside plants from the Tundra.

St. Brigid's Vocational School, County Loughrea 3-28-12

The world is a very big place—on that day it got just a little bit smaller. The concert at St. Brigid's Vocational School in Galway created an instant bond between students who normally share their love of music in very different places, thousands of miles away. That afternoon, they couldn't get on each other's Facebook page fast enough.

Day Five began with a tour of Connemara Marble, and a demonstration on how the famous green marble, unique to Ireland, is used in beautiful jewelry.

Our wonderful guide, Liam, didn't want to pass up an opportunity for the kids to venture out on the beach on the way to the school concert—as long as they didn't track sand on the bus—my kinda guy!

As we pulled into the parking lot of St. Brigid's, the kids couldn't contain their excitement at the special reception from their Irish companions. The concert was magical. Our students were amazing, and their Irish counterparts were thrilled by the American students' performance. BTW, I didn't see one parent chaperone with a dry eye in the place, myself included.

When it was time for the St. Brigid's students to perform, our kids were just as amazed, if not more so, by the wonderful representation of Irish culture in music, song and dance.

After the concert the students had a chance to socialize. They were

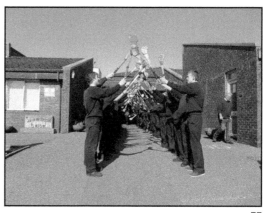

so curious, and wanted to know more about each other on every level. Observing this was so touching. If we just open our eyes, and try to look at the world without blinders, we can see that we really aren't all that different from one another. We can learn so much from our children.

Dublin 3-29-12

With every performance in each different city of Ireland, not only did I learn more about this delightful country, I learned more about these very talented OPRFHS students.

During the evening concert on Day Five, many our our kids' new friends from St. Brigid's came to see them perform in our hotel ballroom. How fitting that the night's concert included a song by The Dubliners—"Night Visiting Song."

On Day Six, as we left Galway and headed to Dublin, our education continued. We stopped at the ancient Monastic site, "Clonmacnoise," nestled along the River Shannon in County Offaly.

This area, known as "The Crossroads of Ireland" was once a major city and place of learning. We must have had the "luck of the Irish" on our side with a picture-perfect day for taking pictures.

As we continued to our final leg of the trip, we stopped for our next performance at Holy Child, an all girls secondary school of 330 students. Once again, we were greeted warmly as if we were dear friends. Our students sang from the heart to their newly found peers.

The young ladies from Holy Child presented us with the gift of song, performing "Cuanla," a traditional Irish folk tune. Several of our senior students had prepared a special arrangement of "Five Years Time" for the concert; the captive audience couldn't wait to hear it.

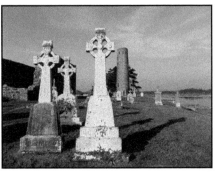

Again I was impressed with how these teens were drawn together through music, making such an important impact in each other's lives.

The Treasures of Dublin 3-30-12

We began with a tour of Dublin Castle, built in 1204 to protect Medieval Dublin.

The original castle was destroyed by fire in 1684 and rebuilt in the 1700's as a Georgian-style castle. With the end of British rule in 1922, the castle's control went to the new Irish Free State Government. Although it is a huge tourist attraction, it remains a working government building—much like our White House.

In the Portrait Gallery, we saw paintings of British Viceroys—some wearing pieces of Ireland's "Crowned Jewels," which were stolen from the castle in 1907, and never found. A reward is still offered for their return, and as our tour guide suggested, "Have at it!"

We saw the very large throne of King George IV, who at some 370 lbs. was England's second largest monarch.

St. Patrick's Hall, one of the oldest rooms in the castle, is used for presidential inaugurations. Across the courtyard, we could to see the only remaining original Medieval structure: the Record Tower and part of the Dublin City wall, and the castle moat below ground.

We were warned not to drop anything into the nasty water, and that's when the drama began. I heard a splash, saw the commotion and realized a student's shoe had fallen in the moat—MY daughter's shoe!

With the help of our guide, a couple sympathetic moms and a broomstick, I was able to retrieve the now disgusting shoe from the slimy water. I proceeded to tell my daughter, "Don't expect a new pair of shoes every time you drop one in a moat!"

With borrowed shoes, we continued on to historic St. Patrick's Cathedral, the largest church in Ireland and the site of our final concert. St. Patrick's was built in the 13th century and has ties to Jonathan Swift's "Gulliver's Travels," and Handel's "Messiah," first sung in1742 at St. Pat's.

After the performance, it was a short walk to Trinity College to see The Book of Kells, a lavishly decorated manuscript of the New Testament, created by Celtic monks in the early 9th century.

We wrapped up our day with a successful shopping excursion in Dublin.

I must be the luckiest chaperone on this trip!

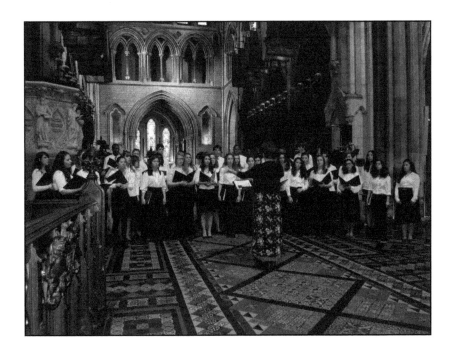

Life Lessons from Ireland 3-31-12

We learn from experience, from our children, and from each other. This perfect trifecta sums up the life lessons I took with me from my Ireland adventure. Remember, I started this trip as a parent chaperone, hoping to spend time with my daughter while exploring a foreign country. I did learn quite a bit about The Emerald Isle; for one, the official color of Ireland is St. Patrick's Blue, not green. Other fun facts:

- The harp is the official symbol of the country—not the Guinness harp, which is opposite of the country's symbol.
- The striking red hair of the Irish people is attributed to the early blending of the blonde Viking men and the black haired, fair Celtic women. Dublin was established as a Viking settlement in the 9th century.
- The city of Dublin gets its name from the Irish words "Dubh Linn" meaning "black pool," referring to the dark colored tidal pool of the nearby River Poddle, which ran under the present site of Dublin Castle (no shoe in the moat jokes, please!)

My travel companions and fellow chaperones came from all walks of life—lawyers, educators, small business owners and performers. They were single parents, blended families, modern families, all somehow making it work. They had a strength I admired, and hearts as big as the country we were visiting.

I learned the most from the students; music is universal and they were here to share that commonality. No matter what drama was going on behind the scenes (they were teens, right?) they were amazing ambassadors, representing our city and country in a most respectable and admirable manner. Every parent would be proud.

A special thanks to one of the girls in my group for making sure I understood the following text speak:

LOL, OMG, LMAO, OTT, GYFO, WTH, JK, ROL, SML, GTHO, TMI, OIC.

A wealth of gratitude goes to Elaine Hlavich, choir director extraordinaire (and my roommate on this trip) for organizing this amazing adventure. The incredible gift of music she gave these 40 students was priceless. The concert at St. Patrick's Cathedral will stay with me always.

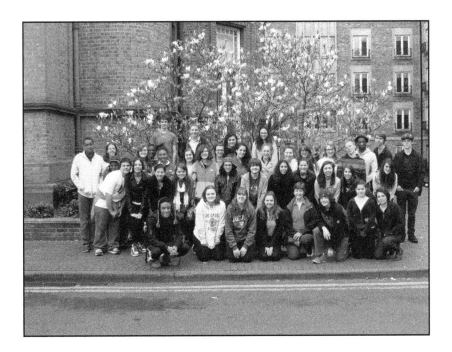

Travel

The Heartland 7-6-12

I love to travel! Of course, if you're reading this book you already know that. My last couple of trips took me overseas in two different continents. I decided this summer vacation would be right here in the good old US of A, visiting states and landmarks that I had never seen before.

Custer State Park is just south of Mt. Rushmore, in the Black Hills of South Dakota. There are miles and miles of scenic trails throughout the 71,000-acre park. We came across lots of pronghorns (similar to an antelope), the fastest land animals in North America, although they stood pretty still for my camera!

We also came across prairie dogs, a wild turkey, and a few high flying hawks. We did not see any bison, probably the wrong time of day, but we did encounter some very friendly burros.

We stopped for a delightful lunch at the Blue Bell Lodge, and yes, they serve bison burgers. We continued winding our way through the park, on roads nestled between the tall ponderosa pines. The views were breathtaking, as the elevation is over 5,000 feet.

The most magnificent site appeared as we went through a narrow one-lane tunnel. As we drove out of the tunnel, we saw in the distance Mt. Rushmore. "O beautiful, for spacious skies...."

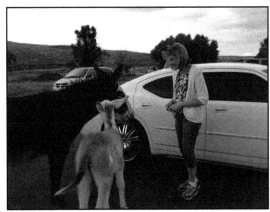

Mt. Rushmore 7-7-12

Our day started with a visit to an American treasure. Mt. Rushmore began as an idea to bring sightseers to the west in the early 1900's; it ended up as so much more!

We took the park ranger tour to get the skinny on the monument. Gutzon Borglum was the sculptor who created this amazing work of art, but he was not the first choice. Chicago artist Lorado Taft was originally asked by historian Doane Robinson to create this masterpiece, but Taft declined due to ailing health.

Borglum chose Mt. Rushmore for the site of his mountain carving because the broad granite wall faced southeast and would receive maximum sunlight, and because granite was a sturdy material that would withhold the test of time. In fact, the estimated erosion rate of Mt. Rushmore is 1 inch every 10,000 years. Spot on Mr. Borglum!

Construction began in 1927. It took 14 years and nearly one million dollars to complete. Actually, it's not really complete. The original design was to show each president from head to waist, but construction was stopped in 1941 due to lack of funding and America's entry into World War II.

You may have also noticed that Lincoln's head is not quite complete—it's missing an ear! Borglum's son Lincoln (named after said president) supervised the completion of the heads after his father's death in 1941, but decided against having another artist add on to it, or change the original work. So, Mt. Rushmore was left as we know it today.

After taking pictures of Mt. Rushmore from every angle imaginable, we took a break and a scenic drive along Needles Highway in nearby Custer State Park—destination, the eye of the needle.

We rounded out the day by returning to Mt. Rushmore for the evening light show featuring a patriotic film, "Freedom—America's Lasting

Legacy," and a tribute to all the service men and women who were in attendance at the show. It was a very moving experience that will stay with me for many years to come.

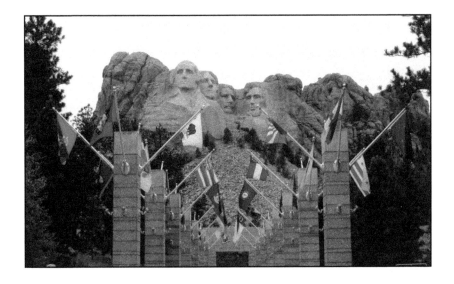

Jewel Cave 7-8-12

We said goodbye to South Dakota, as we hit the road heading west to Sheridan Wyoming, a one night stopping point on the way to Yellowstone National Park.

We decided to do a little sightseeing along the way, and since this was a National Park road trip, we stopped to visit the first cave given National Park status. Jewel Cave is 161 miles long, and still growing, as it is still being explored. Our tour took us 300 feet below the surface, through many caverns and up and down 700 stairs!

When prospector brothers Frank and Albert Michaud made the discovery in 1900, they found a small cave with sparkling crystals, thus the name Jewel Cave. The crystals turned out to be sparkling calcite, which is worth—you guessed it—nothing! The brothers tried but failed to make the cave a tourist attraction. The underground wonder eventually attracted national attention; in 1908 it become part of the National Park System to protect its extraordinary beauty.

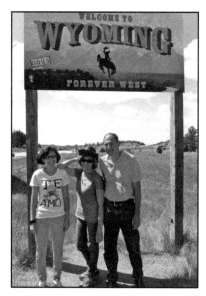

It wasn't until an expedition in 1959 by renowned rock climbers Herb and Jan Conn, that a bigger discovery was made. Over the next 21 years the couple found 65 more miles of this wondrous cave. The mystery continues, however, as experts believe the 161 known miles of Jewel Cave make up only 5% of what lies beneath the Black Hills.

Cody, Wyoming 7-9-12

It must be the hat. I had found my inner cowgirl, and she was not leaving any time soon!

Our road trip continued west from Sheridan to Cody, destination—the Buffalo Bill Historical Center.

We plotted our route and figured it would take close to four hours depending on traffic (just kidding—so used to saying that back home). As we drove, the landscape began to change, and suddenly we found ourselves driving up through forests and mountains.

We were now in Bighorn National Forest, elevation over 8,000 feet. The view was incredible! The land is a history lesson—rock formations of limestone, dolomite and more dating back 500 million years. This truly is God's Country.

We exited Bighorn with a new appreciation of nature's creations and entered the town of Cody, home of the Buffalo Bill Historical Center. If you've ever wanted to learn about the life and times of Buffalo Bill Cody, this is the place to do it. The museum had recently been renovated—it's actually five museums in one, including the original home where William F. Cody spent his early years.

I was most interested in learning more about this legendary figure, so we spent the majority of our time in the Buffalo Bill exhibit. William Cody was given the moniker as a young man when he was hired as a buffalo hunter to supply meat for the rail-

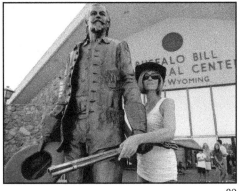

road workers and army personal in Kansas. His skill earned him the nickname, which would eventually be known worldwide. "Buffalo Bill's Wild West" exhibit traveled all over the world, including Chicago for the World's Columbian Exposition in 1893.

With a limited schedule, we still made time to visit the other sections of the museum, including the amazing exhibit on the Plaines Indian Peoples, Western Art, Yellowstone Natural History and Firearms.

As my inner Annie Oakley bade a fond farewell to Buffalo Bill, we continued west to Yellowstone. Yellowstone National Park was the first to receive this designation in 1872. It's easy to see why—its beauty is breathtaking, and its historical and geological significance, overwhelming.

No sooner did we enter the park when we were greeted by roaming bison—several of them along the road, near the geysers, just about everywhere.

Hard to leave—but we had to check into our lodge. Along the way, we made one more stop to admire the beauty and sheer force of the rapids along the Yellowstone River.

Yellowstone National Park 7-10-12

Because there would be less people and more wildlife, we got an early start to Old Faithful. We were not disappointed! Barely 30 minutes on the road and we happened upon a herd of bison. It was awe-inspiring. The biggest clue that animals are approaching: all traffic stops.

We continued south, passing the Lower and Upper Geyser Basins. To see the steam rising from the ground in so many places was almost eerie. In fact, there are more geysers at Yellowstone than anywhere in the world.

Of course the most well known geyser in the world is Old Faithful—conveniently, its eruptions are on a schedule! During our visit, Old Faithful was blowing off steam every 90 minutes or so. We hiked a couple of miles, taking in the sights (and smells) of the many other geysers and sulphur basins in the area.

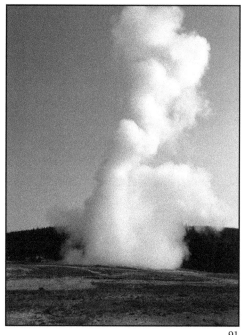

We decided to take the scenic loop back to our lodge. The Continental Divide crossed the road several times—total tourist photo op! Once again, the incredible scenery was worth the drive. The Grand Canyon of Yellowstone offers one of the most beautiful waterfalls we had seen—complete with a rainbow.

Mammoth Hot Springs 7-11-12

We covered so much ground at Yellowstone—it seemed like three days in one. We hit the road early, heading toward Mammoth Hot Springs. We drove past waterfalls, wildlife and a petrified tree, dating back to the Eocene times.

When a chain of volcanoes erupted at this location 50 million years ago, it triggered massive landslides. The rolling mix of ash, water and dirt covered the forest. The silica in the lava flow plugged the living cells in the trees creating a "forest of stone."

The locked gate protects the only remaining petrified tree at Yellowstone. As we continued north, we saw several cars parked along the side of the road. This could mean only one thing—a wildlife sighting! We were in luck—it turned out to be a mother black bear with two cubs. This was a great area to spot black bears; up the road we were treated to yet another.

The scenery changed dramatically as we approached Mammoth Hot Springs. About 50 hot springs are concentrated in this area—the average temperature is 160-degrees! Remember, Yellowstone is sitting over a volcano; in some spots the magma chamber is only five miles from the surface.

As if we hadn't had enough of hot springs and geysers, we left Mammoth to check out the Norris Geyser Basin, another hot spot, the last super volcano at Yellowstone dating back 640-thousand years.

We decided to make the Yellowstone loop complete and visit Old Faithful one more time, just to blow off a little steam! We topped off the evening celebrating my husband Glenn's birthday with "Lava Cake" or "Caldera Cake," as they call it here. The drive back to the lodge at sundown in the rain was a little unnerving, but that's all part of the adventure.

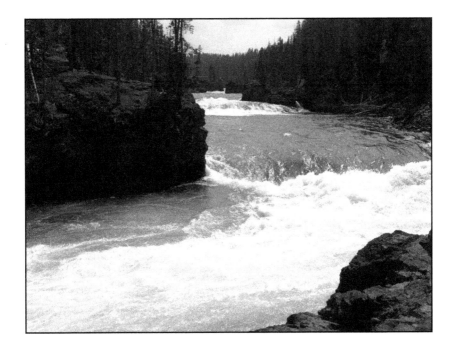

Grand Teton 7-15-12

Had I known that I would see so many amazing things on our Grand National Parks' road trip, I would have given us several more days. Our last two days were spent in Grand Teton National Park.

On the drive south we witnessed another herd of bison. They were so close we could hear them grunt (I think that's the sound they make.) This was our day for wildlife sightings. We took scenic Gull Point Drive adjacent to Yellowstone Lake, and saw a beaver hard at work.

The best photo op just happened upon us when two large elk popped out of the forest and began walking along the side of the road. Absolutely amazing!

As we drove south on Highway 89, 191/287, the majestic mountains peaked up above the forest, waiting to greet us. The snow-capped Tetons were simply breathtaking.

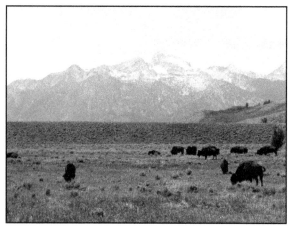

We drove to several overlooks, hoping to see more wildlife. We saw plenty of bison, a couple of pronghorn, but had yet to spot a moose. We made that our mission before we left.

Our last day at Jackson Hole, Wyoming brought another first for me—whitewater rafting! The first half was a scenic float along the Snake River. We were thrilled to see so many bald eagles, as well as pelicans and other wildlife.

The second half of the trip was not so tranquil. Eight miles of white-water rapids! I have to admit, it was exhilarating. I can't believe I was ever nervous.

The best part of the trip came at day's end. We were telling some of the other folks on the whitewater trip about our mission to find a moose. As fortune would have it, they had seen two of these magnificent creatures earlier in the day, "this close to our lodge!" Much to my surprise, the directions they gave us were spot on; and yes, we found our moose!

Life

The Avon Walk for Breast Cancer
2-27-13

No, it was not October—it wasn't even May. We were not surrounded by everything pink—it was February and we were surrounded by snow! Yet for some reason I had recently been asked by numerous organizations to speak at their events as a breast cancer survivor. I am always flattered by these requests. What many of you may not know—the speaking engagements turn out to be as inspirational for me as for the thousands of women and men in the audience. I love the energy, the interaction, and the respect for our mutual journeys.

That being said, I had taken on a new challenge. I signed up for the two day "Avon Walk For Breast Cancer in Chicago" June 1st and 2nd. It was more than just a personal challenge; it had been a way for me to connect with thousands of survivors, friends and family of survivors, and those passionate about helping to find a cure.

I thought long and hard about making this commitment, as it was not an easy task. I trained for the next three months, walking several miles four to five days a week. My biggest concern was not the physical aspect, but the time factor. Then again, my philosophy has always been, I'm at my best when I'm busiest.

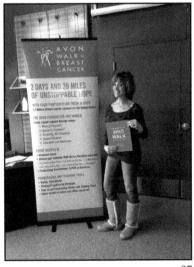

In order to keep myself motivated, I enlisted a partner—my daughter, who was 17 at the time. Sara trained with me as we motivated each other. She helped me document, I helped her fundraise. Together we were unstoppable!

Travel: Rt. 66

The Road Trip of All Road Trips!
7-16-13

The title speaks for itself. Yes, we drove "The Mother Road," Route 66! Just to clarify, my husband drove; my daughter Sara and I navigated "...*from Chicago to LA, more than 2-thousand miles all the way!*"

I got the bug to do this trip last year when our family vacation took us driving through the National Parks of Yellowstone and Grand Teton. Of the eight states that the old Rt. 66 passes through, I had never been to three of them—so many places to explore in the good old US of A.

We left on Saturday July 20th, taking two weeks to leisurely drive cross-country, and then flew back from LA, getting our kicks on Route 66.

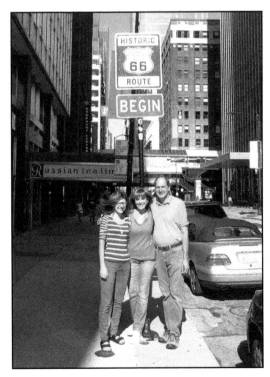

Chicago to Kirkwood, MO 7-20-13

Our first day driving Rt. 66 was filled with surprises around every turn. We started, literally at point zero, in downtown Chicago at Michigan and Adams. We drove down Ogden Avenue, snapping pics along the way.

We spent quite a bit of time on Joliet Road, eventually making our way to Joliet, IL—lots of Blues Brothers sightings there.

In Wilmington we found the first of many larger-than-life fiberglass statues—the Gemini Giant at the (now closed) Launching Pad Drive-In.

Do not pass go, do not collect $200—go directly to jail! In Gardner, the two-cell jail built in 1906 is a popular photo op.

More photo ops presented themselves in Odell at a restored Standard Sinclair station built in 1932. It is now an information center and souvenir shop.

My biggest surprise came as we drove into Pontiac. Mayor Bob Russell and many others in town were waiting for us at the Rt. 66 Museum—they even put up welcome signs.

Two hours late, we hit the road again. We had to stop at Funks Grove to try the much talked about maple "sirup." So glad I did, it was pure and delicious.

Time passed much too quickly to take in all the sites on my list We continued on to St. Louis, driving over the Mighty Mississippi to Kirkwood, ready for a well-deserved night's rest.

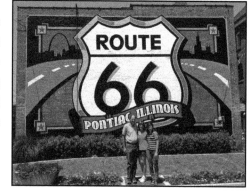

Kirkwood, MO to Tulsa, OK 7-21-13

Day Two along the Mother Road began with a stop at the Rt. 66 State Park in Eureka, Missouri. This 419-acre park along the Meramec River has several inviting trails, but we were more interested in the Visitor Center Museum, filled with Rt. 66 memorabilia.

The rolling hills of the Show Me State were quite scenic, varying from vast greenery to the many Rt. 66 roadside attractions. In Springfield, we came across a giant paper cup. Actually, it was part of the architecture of the building that housed the Solo Cup Company. This particular plant closed in 2011.

Another historic site, Dale's Barbershop in Joplin originated in 1929 as a Shamrock gas station. It was converted into a barbershop in1962 until the owner retired in 2004.

As we approached the Kansas state line, we stopped for a quick pic at the Hogs and Hot Rods Saloon. Back in the day, Kansas used to be a dry state, making this 1925 state line honky-tonk a popular destination.

Kansas has the shortest stretch of Rt. 66 of all the states—only 13 miles—but we found plenty to see. The Eisler Brothers Old Riverton Store is a throwback to the general store days of yesteryear—complete with pink flamingos on the lawn.

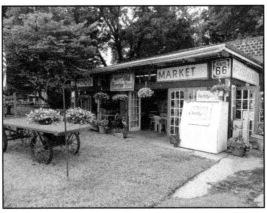

The Rainbow Arch Bridge, built in 1926, is on the national Register of Historic Places, and you can still drive over it.

Entering Oklahoma, Rt. 66 took us through Quapaw, once a booming mining town as depicted in one of the many Quapaw murals.

In Miami (pronounced my-am-uh, from the Native American tribe), we saw the Coleman Theater. Built in 1929 in the Spanish Revival style, it was a vaudeville and movie palace. It remains open to this day.

After traveling over 425 miles through three states, we were about to hit the halfway mark on the way to Amarillo, TX.

Tulsa, OK to Amarillo, TX 7-23-13

For those of you preparing for a road trip of your own along The Great American Highway, a word of advice—however much time you think you'll need to drive it, DOUBLE IT! Who knew Oklahoma was such a big state? Another jam-packed day, we logged more than 380 miles along the Mother Road.

Leaving Tulsa, there were many reminders that we were in the Oil Capital of The World. The Ozark Trail alignment featured old, rusted oil tanks, symbols of the oil boom during the heyday of Rt. 66.

We drove along American's Main Street through many small towns filled with former gas stations-turned-cafes, shops, or simply tourist attractions. We stopped for lunch in Arcadia Oklahoma at Pops, a landmark diner and gas station with over 500 kinds of sodas, and a 66-foot-tall soda bottle out front!

It took quite a bit longer than we thought to drive through Oklahoma—we actually veered back on the interstate for a bit to save some time. Closer to the Texas border, we tipped our hat to Will Rogers at the landmark plaque dedicating Rt. 66 as Will Rogers Highway.

We took pictures at the state line. We saw the stunning 1936 art deco design of the U-Drop Inn in Shamrock, TX. We marveled at the purposely-crooked Leaning Tower of Britten, designed to catch a tourist's eye and get them to stop in Groom, TX.

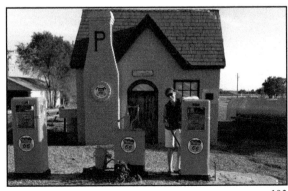

Shortly before 9:00 pm, we pulled into Amarillo to catch a few zzzzz's, but first, dinner at The Big Texan Restaurant, home of the Free 72 oz. steak (if you can eat it in an hour!). Imagine their confusion when my daughter and I ordered a 6 oz. filet—to share between us.

Amarillo, TX to Santa Fe, NM
7-24-13

Our Rt. 66 adventure took an artistic turn. They say everything is big in Texas, right? That especially held true for the larger-than-life art in Amarillo. Cadillac Ranch is not a ranch, but an art installation consisting of 10 Cadillacs, nose down, painted daily by touristy artists, like ourselves.

Not too far from Amarillo, we hit a milestone in Adrian—the halfway point! Only 1,139 miles to go. We marked the occasion at The MidPoint Cafe, "Home of the Ugly Pie Crust." Yes, the pie and the crust were delicious!

After a mere 22 miles, we entered New Mexico, and that's when the driving got a little hairy.

Once we got on the stretch of Rt. 66 that shared the interstate, the surroundings took on a completely different attitude—serene, majestic, inviting. We took the pre-1937 route that brought us into Santa Fe, arriving with enough time to take in a little sightseeing before dinner. We visited San Miguel Mission, said to be the oldest standing church in the U.S., built in 1610. Across the street was the oldest house in Santa Fe (and according to their literature, in the U.S.), built in 1646.

We walked through town at dusk, and while many of the wonderful shops and boutiques were closed, the park was alive with a summer concert. What a great way to end the day.

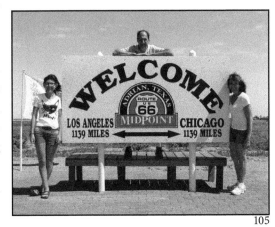

Santa Fe, NM to Albuquerque, NM
7-25-13

Santa Fe, New Mexico had to be one of the most charming cities I'd ever seen. From the historic adobe architecture to the hundreds of art galleries, it was a feast for the eyes.

We began our day with a visit to the Georgia O'Keeffe Museum, which houses the largest number of works in the world from this iconic artist. I have been a Georgia O'Keeffe aficionado for as long as I can remember—especially since my world class art photographer uncle, Malcolm Varon, had an opportunity to spend time with O'Keeffe, taking pictures of her, as well as her artwork.

Imagine my surprise, and delight not only seeing Uncle Malcolm's name in the credits of a short movie on O'Keeffe, but also on several prints, books and calendars in the gift shop. So proud to be related to this incredibly talented photographer.

We continued to enjoy this picture-perfect day walking around the plaza, taking in the sites and sounds, lunching at an outdoor cafe.

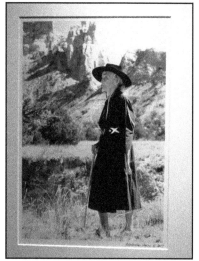

We got back on the road, headed to Albuquerque—our next stop on Rt. 66. The bright sunshine was quickly replaced with clouds—ominous clouds as we continued south. Radar showed some fast-moving storms, along with flash flood alerts! We decided to stay on I-25 most of the way, just in case. Fortunately the heavy storms missed us, and we made our way safely to Albuquerque, back on Rt. 66.

Exploring Albuquerque 7-26-13

It was our 6th day traveling Rt. 66. We were averaging over 300 miles a day, but this day logged only 78. We spent it driving in and around Albuquerque.

Our first stop was the Sandia Mountains located within the Cibola National Forest. We explored a bit first, checking out the ski slopes and hiking trails, which were dipping in and out of the clouds. Quite an experience!

After a break from the high altitude, we ventured west to the Petroglyph National Monument. This National Park contains more than 20,000 images carved in stone—some recognizable as animals or people, others more mysterious. Archeologists estimate most of the images were made 400 to 700 years ago by the ancestors of today's Native people. Some images, however, could be some 2,000 to 3,000 years old.

In our limited amount of time we were able to hike three short trails and see dozens of petroglyphs. One can only imagine the significance these images represented hundreds of years ago, perhaps thousands.

Our day ended with dinner in Albuquerque's Old Town at a charming Mexican-American restaurant. The vibrant colors of the sunset over the mountains were just a taste of things to come as we left the "Land of Enchantment" and continued our road trip west.

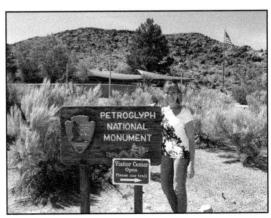

Albuquerque, NM to Flagstaff, AZ
7-27-13

Another 370-plus miles on the odometer as we bade farewell to Albuquerque; destination, Flagstaff, AZ.

The morning started out in a GRAND way, crossing the Rio Grande! We passed plenty of Rt. 66 signage—some new, many vintage, as the scenery became less and less residential.

A stop near the town of Thoreau was a must to snap a pic at the Continental Divide marker. Wouldn't you know it, there was a HUGE souvenir shop across the road to mark the occasion.

By now we were ready for lunch and decided to stop in Gallup. We were using this incredible app, "Road Trip 66" to help guide us. One recommendation was Earl's Family Restaurant. As we pulled up, the parking lot was jammed; a very good sign.

Native American artisans sold handmade crafts, both inside the restaurant and outside. Sara found something special, for someone special. We even had a friendly chat with owner Ralph Richards, giving us some helpful tips for our continuing journey.

As we crossed the border into Arizona, the scenery changed again. We saw wild horses taking shelter from the heat in a tunnel under I-40. We saw "Fort Courage" in the form of yet another souvenir shop, modeled after the '60s sit-com "F-Troop."

The highpoint of the day was a two-fer, courtesy of Mother Nature: Petrified Forest National Park and the Painted Desert. I had never seen anything like this and will hold on to these incredibly beautiful images for as long as humanly possible.

About half way between the Painted Desert and the Petrified Forest, we found "Newspaper Rock," so named because of the thousands of petroglyphs—images scratched on stone—that were made by native people hundreds, even thousands of years ago.

Appropriately enough, there was an old model car on a spot dedicated was to where Rt. 66 had cut through the park. To the left of that, we saw the line of old telephone poles that still marked the roadbed of Historic Rt. 66.

I could have spent days, rather than hours capturing the magnificent structures and vibrant hues, but with the storms looming and the temperature dropping, we knew we were on borrowed time.

The rains became heavy—even blinding for a stretch, but we were not going to let that stop us from visiting the "Take It Easy" corner, made famous by the Eagles 1972 hit song. I just love pop culture!

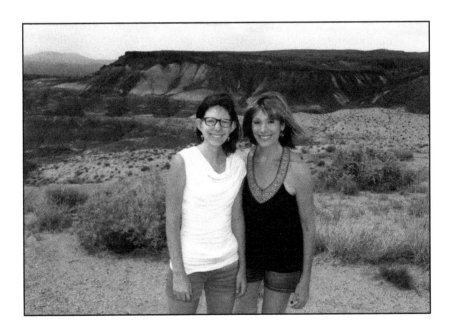

Flagstaff, AZ to Needles, CA
7-28-13

Have you ever had a day that felt like three jammed into one? Well that was our day on Rt. 66 from Flagstaff, AZ to Needles, CA; and I meant that in a good way. We started with a late breakfast at the Galaxy Diner—a '50s style eatery with great food to go with the retro decor.

Our first stop after breakfast was along Brannigan Park Road in Belmont, AZ, in Kaibab National Forest, which is said to be the highest point along Rt. 66, elevation 7,412 ft.

The next stop was Williams, where we had the option to take the train on a side trip to the Grand Canyon. Since we had already seen that magnificent site on previous vacations, we opted to walk through Williams, which has become a mecca for all things Rt. 66.

All that sightseeing (and shopping) worked up an appetite; good thing the Road Kill Cafe in Seligman was just a short drive away. Yes, the food was DELICIOUS; no, it wasn't really road kill!

We had hoped to take a side trip down Diamond Creek Road to see the bottom of the Grand Canyon at the Colorado River, but due to the heavy rains over the past several days, the road was flooded and impassable. Instead, we stopped at the General Store in Hackberry and found a treasure trove of Rt. 66 memorabilia and souvenirs.

Entering Kingman, the scenery changed once again, from forest to a quaint town set against a backdrop of rugged mountains. No shortage of Rt. 66 history here, from the welcoming water towers to the train depot-turned museum.

Driving through the mountains, the rains moved in and here's where things got interesting. Fortunately my husband, Glenn, was an exceptional driver—and the rain let up.

As we approached the town of Oatman, we were greeted by the infamous burros. Oatman, AZ was a gold mining town in the early 1900's with more than 3,500 residents. It's now described as a "living ghost town" with perhaps 100 residents. But for visitors along Rt. 66, this throwback to the Old West is a must-see.

The drive leaving Oatman was just as scenic, especially since we had sun glistening from the mountaintops, and a rainbow to boot!

There were many times we felt like we had the road to ourselves. And out there, in the desert, in the middle of nowhere, there was still a reminder that we were traveling on the most historic stretch of roadway in America.

We were just 22 miles from our stop for the night, Needles, CA. We followed the old Rt. 66 alignment as we crossed into California, but somehow this road was no longer an option; it was filled with rocks and was impassable!

We shifted to the interstate, and within minutes found ourselves approaching the town of Needles, so named for its pointed mountain peaks. We paused for a picture, and paused for a night's rest.

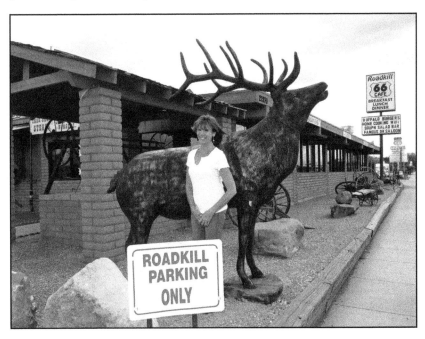

Needles, CA to Barstow, CA
7-29-13

As we began the 9th day of our Rt. 66 journey, we thought we would, as the song says, "Take it Easy," and only travel the 155 miles from Needles to Barstow.

With a high of 105-degrees predicted for our drive through the desert, we loaded up with ice and water and hit the road. One thing I noticed driving the Mother Road through California there were very few street signs marking Historic Rt. 66. Instead, the iconic shields were on the pavement itself.

Driving through the Mojave Desert was hot—our car thermometer was proof—but that did not take away from the majestic beauty of the mountains in the distance.

As this was monsoon season in the southwest desert, we found ourselves driving into threatening-looking storm systems with severe lightening in the distance. Fortunately the storms stayed to the north allowing us to partake in the "Rock Art" along the railroad berm just east of the town of Amboy. There was a several mile stretch decorated with initials, greetings, signatures—all spelled out in rocks.

Our next stop was a National Natural Landmark—The Amboy Crater and Lava Field. The crater is an extinct 250 ft. high volcanic cinder cone that lies within a 27-square mile lava field in the Mojave Desert. One can hike to the top of the cone, but with temps topping out at 108-degrees, instead, we chose to take pictures under the shade of the visitors' lookout.

One of the most delightful things about driving Rt. 66 were the tourists we met along the way. The people in every town we visited were more than hospitable and all had stories to tell. Travelers like ourselves, they conveyed the same amount of enthusiasm and wonder as they ventured cross country on this historic highway.

112

Roy's Motel and Cafe was one of only a few left along this stretch of 66 in the desert and came with an interesting story. Amboy was a railroad town before Rt. 66 was built.

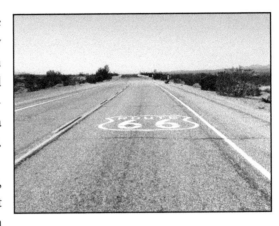

When the highway, and the subsequent travelers came through during the Great Depression, Roy Crowl opened a diner with great success.

When I-40 rerouted traffic around Amboy, the town died. (As a traffic specialist, it always fascinates me to see how new highway construction can affect the lives of the local community.)

Fast-forward to 2005—Albert Okura, owner of the Juan Pollo Restaurants bought the entire town, and was said to be in the process of restoring many structures. It was looking good as we drove by.

Our final stop was the Bagdad Cafe in Newberry Springs, which was the inspiration and location for the 1988 film, "Bagdad Cafe."

Barstow, CA to Santa Monica, CA
7-30-13

I woke up with mixed emotions. For the past nine days, I had been looking so forward to reaching our final stop on Rt. 66, and now that it was rapidly approaching I didn't want the journey to end.

Coffee in hand, we pulled out of Barstow on our way to Santa Monica. I wanted to capture as many images as I could of the iconic road as we drove west, mountains beckoning.

In the town of Helandale, a rather unusual sight popped up, seemingly out of nowhere! Elmer Long's Bottle Cactus Ranch was filled with trees made of bottles—hundreds of them! Long created this unusual display after inheriting a huge bottle collection from his father. Quite a colorful spot in the middle of the desert!

The next town gave us an opportunity to do some antiquing at the Oro Grande Antique Station. I found some interesting items, but I thought they would go over the weight limit in my suitcase, so I abandoned the idea.

More movie history in Victorville—a stop at Emma Jean's Holland Burger Cafe—great Rt. 66 road food, and was featured in the film "Kill Bill." What more would you want in a cafe?

Heading south between Angeles National Forest and San Bernadino National Forest, the scenery was breathtaking against the clear blue sky.

More fun sights approached on Foothill Boulevard—The Wigwam Village Motel in Rialto, and Bono's Giant Orange Stand in Fontana. The motel is open; the juice stand has closed.

The city of Rancho Cucamonga had many beautiful Rt. 66 displays, both alongside and above the roadway.

Next town over, the Madonna Of The Trail paid tribute to the pioneer women who traveled west with their husbands and children. From serious to surreal—more towering fiberglass as Chicken Boy looked down on us from a rooftop in LA.

For lunch, we decided on a recommendation from the "Road Trip 66" app we had been following—Mom's Tamales in Lincoln Heights. All I can say is WOW! Best tamales I'd had outside of Mexico—seriously.

Beyond Los Angeles, Rt. 66 follows Santa Monica Blvd. We passed several famous sights: The Hollywood Forever Cemetery—the final resting place of many famous actors, directors and producers; The Troubadour, where many musicians and performers got their start.

At long last, we hit the end point of Rt. 66 at Santa Monica Blvd and Ocean Avenue, where we received a certificate from the Santa Monica Convention & Visitor's Bureau for making the 2,448-mile journey from Chicago.

It was bittersweet, but the experience will stay with me for a lifetime. As we know, life is a journey, not a destination—this was just part of the journey.

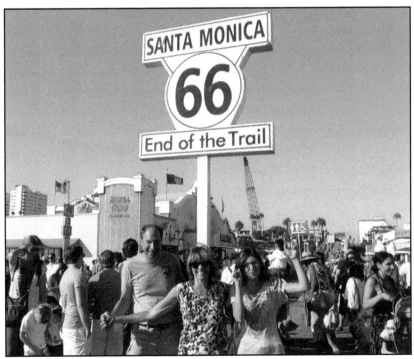

Santa Monica, CA Back Home to Chicago, IL 8-4-13

No matter how amazing the trip, it's always good to come home. Such was the case with our Rt. 66 journey—home, safe and sound, basking in the wonderful memories. There is, however, a postscript.

For those of you who are interested in motoring along the Mother Road, I've put together a timeline—how many miles per day, and where we stayed.

We decided to rent a vehicle (mini-van) and fly back so we could take our time over a two-week period. I spent time researching the route, using two very helpful tools—the website "Historic Route 66" http://www.historic66.com/, and an app, "Road Trip 66."

The website gave us an idea of what we were in for ahead of time, but the app was my main form of information and navigation throughout the trip. It gave us the entire route, old alignments and new; about 97% of the time it was spot-on. Pretty impressive, because the infamous route no longer exists, it turns out there really are no maps of Rt. 66.

Day 1—We drove 309 miles from Chicago to Kirkwood, MO and stayed at the Best Western, 1200 S. Kirkwood Rd. With all the stops along the way (and 2 hours in Pontiac, IL) this took 10 hours.

Day 2—We drove 431 miles from Kirkwood, MO to Tulsa, OK and stayed at the Campbell Hotel, 2600 E. 11th St. This restored boutique hotel was built in 1927 and is on the National Register of Historic Places. This was our longest driving day. We actually had to get off Rt. 66 and take I-40 part of the way to make up some time. (Kind of misjudged this one a bit—even with the Interstate it took 11 hours.)

Day 3—We drove 402 miles from Tulsa, OK to Amarillo, TX and stayed at The Big Texan Motel, 7701 I-40 East. Again, another L O N G driving day—11 hours. Never having been to these states, I didn't realize how long a drive it would be, particularly with stops along the way.

Day 4—We drove 310 miles from Amarillo, TX to Santa Fe, NM and stayed at the Santa Fe Sage Inn, 725 Cerrillos Rd. This drive was lovely and short, comparatively speaking. We rolled into town at 3:30 pm. Never having been to the state of New Mexico, we opted to stay one night in Santa Fe and two nights in Albuquerque. In hindsight, I would have done the opposite. Santa Fe is such a charming town, an artists' town with history and character. Loved it!

Day 5—A short 77-mile drive from Santa Fe, NM to Albuquerque, NM. We stayed at The Hotel Blue, 717 Central Ave. This hotel had an unusual feel to it; no pictures on the walls. But it was clean and it had Tempurpedic beds. Good enough for me. Stayed here two nights.

Day 7—We drove 368 miles from Albuquerque, NM to Flagstaff, AZ. This was a long day because we spent hours driving through the Painted Desert and Petrified Forest National Park. SO worth it! Also hit some major storms (monsoon season) and rolled into the Radisson Woodlands Hotel, 1175 W. Rt. 66 around 7:30 pm.

 Day 8—We spent this day driving across Arizona—243 miles—to Needles, CA. We stayed at the Best Western Colorado River Inn. To make sure we had water and ice, and the car was in good shape, we decided to stop there before spending a day driving in the Mojave Desert.

Day 9—We drove 161 miles through the desert from Needles, CA to Barstow, CA. We took our time, drank plenty of fluids and arrived at the Rodeway Inn, 1261 E. Main St. around 3:00 pm. This gave us time to repack, do some laundry and prepare for the upcoming week.

Day 10—It was only 168 miles from Barstow, CA to Santa Monica, CA and the end of Rt. 66, but once we got into the LA traffic grid it seemed like it took FOREVER. We finally made it to the Santa Monica Pier around 5:00 pm. After we took the celebratory pictures, had dinner and just enjoyed the ocean view, we checked into the Doubletree by Hilton at 4th and Olympic, just "off" Rt. 66—the only hotel that wasn't located exactly on the historic route. We stayed there four nights, visiting family and friends before flying home on Day 14.

One last bit of parting advice: if you do decide to tackle this baby, give yourself MORE time than you think you'll need. Even with all my planning, I could have easily used another week, and there were still things I wouldn't have been able to see.

Good luck, and happy motoring!

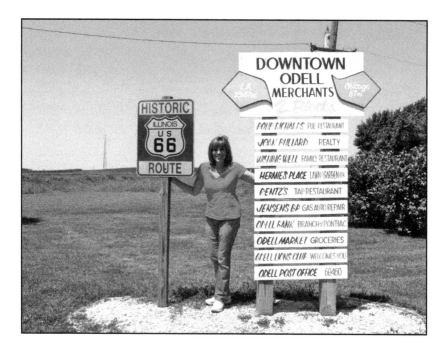

Travel: New York City

NYC 3-22-14

After surviving the most brutal winter I could remember, I should have been spending "Spring Break" in the most tropical climate. Instead, I was heading to New York, on my final trip as a school chaperone—bittersweet, I know.

I felt the same way when Sara decided not to continue with Girl Scouts, after having been her leader for 8 years. In just a few hours I would be joining more than 70 Oak Park & River Forest High School Choir students and chaperones on a weeklong trip to New York City! The students would be performing at several locations, as well as seeing several Broadway shows. Each chaperone was responsible for a group of 5 to 6 students during show time, as well as free time.

Here's where it got interesting...my group of students was comprised of Sara...AND 5 BOYS! How did this happen? I don't know, but honestly it turned out to be a blessing in disguise! These young men wanted to take in the sights and sounds of the Big Apple during their free time, as opposed to say, shopping. They were so serious about our group scheduling fun activi-

ties, that they created a group Facebook page so we could more easily make plans during our "free time." Impressive.

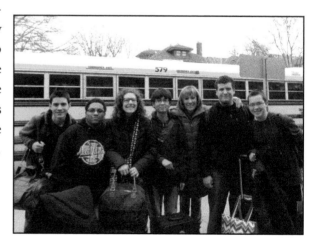

Midtown 3-23-14

The past two days had been a whirlwind! It started Saturday afternoon with a farewell dinner at the school and some 60 students who could barely contain their excitement.

My group, affectionately known as "Sara and The Boys," had been among the first on the bus to Union Station. Still bursting with energy, they found ways to occupy themselves waiting for Amtrak's Lake Shore Limited, which not surprisingly departed an hour behind schedule.

By the time we had rolled out of Chicago, it was close to 11:00 pm. As tired as we were, those of us who were lucky enough to drift off to dreamland didn't get more than a handful of hours of sleep.

Speaking strictly for myself, definitely a "Motrin Moment." That Sunday morning brought us through Cleveland Ohio, past Erie Pennsylvania, then stopping in Buffalo New York, where a fresh snowstorm reminded us that while the calendar said spring, winter still had an icy grip on much of the country.

Eventually, the sun broke through and we were treated to a very scenic train ride through upstate New York. By 6:30 pm, after more than 20 hours on the train, the excitement began to mount as we approached our final destination—Penn Station.

For most of the students, this had been their first experience in "The City That Never Sleeps." I took my group to the Brooklyn Diner, for some gi-normous sandwiches!

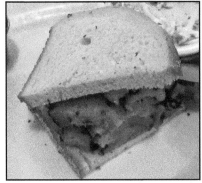

On the walk back to our hotel, we couldn't help but stop for a quick tourist moment near Times Square.

Uptown 3-26-14

Our first full day in New York began with a quick breakfast and subway ride Uptown for the students' first performance at St. John the Divine.

After the performance, we had a few hours of free time. Several of the guys in my group had requested a visit to Nintendo World. They checked out the latest video games; I checked my email!

After that grueling game, it was time for some gruel. You know the saying…when in Rome—so I took them to a Kosher Deli. I felt the need to top off all that pastrami with some chocolate—how convenient, the M & M store was just a few blocks away.

For dinner, the entire group met at Da Nico Ristorante in Little Italy. A charming place with authentic food in a historic neighborhood.

Me being me I couldn't end the day right then and there—so I took my group to see "Avenue Q." Of course they loved it! Of course with my group consisting of my daughter and five teen guys, no surprise there.

Yes, it had been a full day and a late night. Yes I was getting them up VERY early the next morning for a big surprise. I guess that's why they call it "The city that doesn't sleep!"

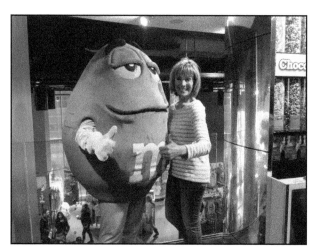

Downtown, Uptown, and Midtown Manhattan 3-27-14

O ur second full day in NYC was full of surprises. My group had a very early wake-up call. We had to be at the stage door of the Good Morning America studios by 6:45 to see the show from "behind the scenes."

My group already knew the GMA visit was in the plans—they didn't know we'd be part of the local "talk-back" with ABC7 Chicago. Luck was on our side, and my group of six not only got to stand on the set behind Robin Roberts, but they also got to sing to her and to all of Chicagoland from New York!

We stayed for the entire two-hour show, which included special guest Diana Nyad, and the band Karmin.

Once the show wrapped, we continued with our ambitiously planned day, heading downtown on the subway to see the 9/11 Memorial.

We had to wait in a long security line to get in, but everyone understood. There was strained sunshine, with a bone-chilling wind, which seemed appropriate during this emotional, yet powerful visit.

The Memorial was beautiful, with two large cascading fountain pools marking the locations where the Twin Towers stood. The new Towers were magnificent, like a phoenix rising with resilience. I wasn't the only one to shed a tear.

Our day continued on an upbeat note, literally, as we took the subway Uptown to the Church of

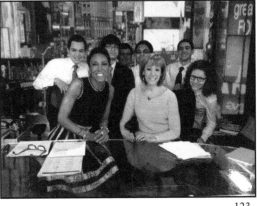

the Blessed Sacrament for the students' next concert. Another impressive performance.

My Uncle Malcolm Varon, a native New Yorker, came to see the concert and then gave our group a brief tour of Central Park. I say brief, because it was SO COLD and brutally windy, even the boys were complaining they needed to get out of the elements!

We wrapped up our day with another Broadway musical, "Matilda," at the Shubert Theatre.

Broadway 3-28-14

Sleeping in had been a good thing. Our first two days were so full, it felt like a week had gone by. Our day started with the students' final concert of the trip, at Madison Sculpture Garden on Madison Avenue near 57th.

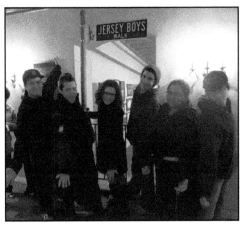

We had some early afternoon free time after the performance; the boys grabbed some lunch, Sara and I snuck in a little shopping.

Our next stop—a matinee of "Jersey Boys." I was so excited to share this experience with my group, as most hadn't seen it—plus I had scored some pretty sweet seats—3rd row orchestra!

I don't know if I was over-tired, over-scheduled or just absent-minded, but I could have sworn the show time was 3:00 pm. When we showed up at 2:45 and no one was in the lobby, I had a really bad feeling! The show had started at 2:00!! I was SO UPSET with myself, I couldn't hide my disappointment. The kids, on the other hand, took the high road, and were so kind and appreciative, it just reaffirmed my assessment of how special my group of students had been. Plus, they still LOVED the show (minus the first 45 minutes).

Next stop—dinner at Juniors—more yummy New York deli-style cuisine in a fun, sit-down setting.

Then, it was time to get ready for our evening event, "La Boheme" at the Metropolitan Opera House at Lincoln Center. The evening temperatures had become bitterly cold with wind gusts of up to 50 mph! I made an executive decision—no walking to the subway that night—we were cabbing it.

The opera was lovely, but I can assure you, with such long, full days, there were many heavy eyelids during the three-hour performance—mine included. It didn't take long to fall fully asleep once we got back to the hotel.

Liberty Island 3-29-14

Hard to believe it was our last full day in NYC—the week had just flown by. Making the most of our precious time, we started out on a morning rush hour subway ride (and you thought the CTA was crowded) to Battery Park.

From there we caught the ferry to see the Statue of Liberty. We had plenty of opportunities to take pictures, as the security lines were long, even with reservations.

The wait to visit Lady Liberty was worth it. Seeing the magnificent torch reaching into a clear blue sky, one could only imagine what thoughts of freedom and opportunity filled the minds of the millions of immigrants as they approached, searching for the "American Dream."

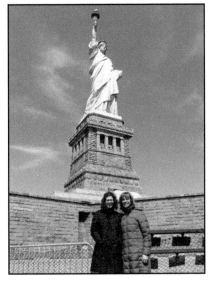

My group of seven toured the museum, climbed the 215 steps from the lobby to the top of the pedestal, caught our breath and captured breathtaking pictures.

The visit wouldn't have been complete without a stop at Ellis Island. At the time this historic National Monument was open on a limited basis only, due to the extensive damage caused by Hurricane Sandy. It was still worth a visit to see the Great Hall, and look at a nearly one hundred year old ship's registry. An amazing piece of American history.

As tired as we were, we forged on to meet with the entire group of 70 students and chaperones at the top of the Empire State Building.

Marveling in its 'art deco' style, we delighted in taking magnificent pictures from the observatory. It was the world's tallest building from 1931 to 1973—CHICAGO CONNECTION—guess what building beat it out as the world's tallest in 1974? The Sears Tower, which became the Willis Tower.

To complete the day, we went back to the theatre district for an 8:00 p.m. performance of "Pippin" at the Music Box Theatre.

Travel: Southern United Kingdom

A Virtual Voyage 7-31-14

Let's wax nostalgic on my next virtual vacation as I set off on a won-drous adventure "across the pond" touring southern England. As if that weren't fabulous enough, I would be traveling with my daughter Sara, just the two of us. This was her graduation gift before she headed off to college next month.

During my 25+ years at ABC7, many of you have watched Sara grow up—here's the nostalgic part—and during that time she has become an incredible traveler!

She took her first cruise before she was two; at four, she was climbing pyramids in Mexico!

At six, Sara had accompanied my Mom and me on a trip to Spain—three generations in our mother country (my heritage is Sephardic.) At

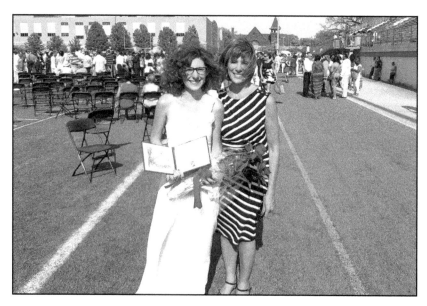

10, Sara was sightseeing through ancient Greece; at 12 she experienced the glaciers of Alaska.

I took her to President Obama's first inauguration—we explored the Holy Land together with members of our congregation.

I chaperoned a high school choir trip to Ireland, and back in the states we took road trips to our national parks and the entire stretch of Rt. 66. Sara's 18th birthday was a destination party to the "Happiest Place on Earth."

On this adventure, I'll share our discoveries in London and many other historic places in the UK.

We arrived at Heathrow Airport on a Monday. A special thanks to my friends on social media for suggestions and advice that made this trip so memorable.

One more thing—a heartfelt thanks to my incredibly understanding husband for giving Sara and I this special bonding time while he stayed at home. Besides, someone had to watch the dogs, right?

Across The Pond 8-4-14

Hello, London! We made it across the pond in less than eight hours—with less than four hours of sleep. Didn't matter—local time 8:45 a.m., we pushed through, checked into our hotel and connected with a friend. In spite of our jet lag, he most graciously took us on a quick walking tour. We started by taking the "tube" to what has to be one of the most touristy streets in the area—but hey, we're tourists, right?

We stopped to pose for a quick pic in front of Abbey Road Studio and another quick pic in front of one of Sir Paul's homes.

As we made our way to lunch, we walked past some beautiful architecture in this affluent part of town, Sticking with the tourist theme, Sara and I both enjoyed a tasty plate of fish 'n' chips.

After a great meal, the jet lag really started to kick it. It was time to head back to the hotel to rest. A most sincere thank you to our special friend and incredible host, Fred Weintraub, for starting our UK trip on the right foot—or is that the left foot—everything here is backwards.

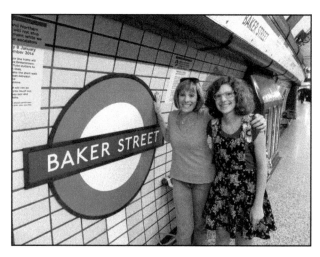

Buckingham Palace 8-5-14

This day was one right out of the history books. We began with a bus tour through the streets of London—each structure more impressive than the last. We saw the original Ritz Hotel, which opened its doors in May of 1906. We passed by Berkeley Square, where a spectacular Chihuly glass sculpture was bursting with color.

We drove past Piccadilly Circus, described by our tour guide as the "Times Square" of London. We gazed at the beauty of Trafalgar Square, a landmark in Westminster, London, where all types of special events are held. (You may recall a *small* wedding with those lovebirds Will and Kate.)

Our first stop was St. Paul's Cathedral, a major London landmark. Built between 1675 and 1710 and designed by Sir Christopher Wren, its dome is the second largest in the world. In fact, Wren is buried in the crypt in the cathedral's lower level, as is Lord Nelson of the Battle of Trafalgar fame, and the Duke of Wellington, a hero in the Battle of Waterloo. More recently, St. Paul's was where Charles, Prince of Wales, was married to Lady Diana Spencer. No photographs were allowed inside the cathedral. Take my word for it; it was beyond magnificent.

As we continued to our next destination, we passed more incredible landmarks—the iconic Big Ben along the River Thames, and the Shard, a modern 87-story, glass-clad pyramid shaped tower.

And then, the moment we had been waiting for! As our group began to walk down The Mall, we heard sirens and saw two black sedans. We looked closely and saw Prince William in the back seat of the first vehicle. That was as close to royalty as I'll ever get—and that's pretty good.

As we approached Buckingham Palace, we were lucky enough to see several parts of the pageantry that made up the Changing of the Guard.

After all that sightseeing, Sara and I were ready to shop. Being the transit-savvy gals that we were, we took our Oyster cards (think Ventra) and hopped on the double-decker 414 to Harrods. Ok, this department store is like Neiman's, Saks, Macy's, and Bloomingdales all wrapped into one—on steroids. They handed out maps, so you wouldn't get lost. We didn't get lost—maybe my cash did! We stopped for tea and scones, made one last trip for gifts, and made our way through the London rush hour. (This traffic specialist admits to being thrown off balance by the drivers on the opposite side of the streets.)

It was such a beautiful evening that we decided to walk back (and work off those scones and clotted cream). We strolled past lovely parks and unique monuments and a street filled with vintage restaurants that reminded me were SO not in the states.

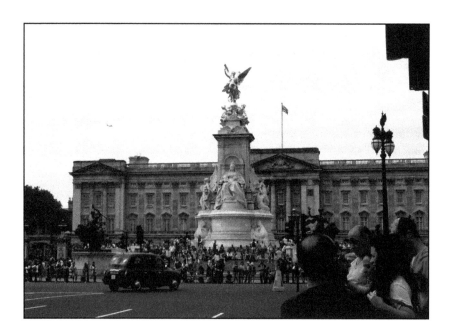

Stratford-Upon-Avon 8-6-14

As we departed England's capital, we finally got some of that rainy weather London is known for. We were on our way to the birthplace of the greatest playwright of all time—but first, a couple of historic stops along the way.

We began our journey back in the 15th century with a visit to Hampton Court Palace & Garden—150 acres along the River Thames, whose most well known resident was Henry VIII.

Our next stop went back in time even further—to Oxford, the oldest University in the English-speaking world, dating back to 1096. The University is made up of 38 colleges; famous Oxonians included 26 British Prime Ministers, at least 30 international leaders, 50 Nobel Prize winners, and 120 Olympic medal winners. We toured, we shopped, and ate meat pies for lunch before heading to our final destination.

Minutes before arriving at the home of William Shakespeare, we made a quick stop at the childhood home of his future wife, Ann Hathaway. The charming cottage was a thatched farmhouse with picturesque gardens right out of a storybook.

We easily spent the most time at our final stop, Shakespeare's Birthplace in Stratford Upon Avon, a lovely town brimming with history. Shakespeare's parents, John and Mary, were wealthy enough to own the largest house on Henley Street. They had eight children there, and the home also doubled as a workshop for Shakespeare's father's glove making business.

When John Shakespeare died, William inherited the house. When Shakespeare died in 1616, he left the house to his eldest daughter, Susanna. It is now owned by the Birthplace Trust to share with visitors from all over the world.

What better place to enjoy a performance of the Bard's work.

I don't think we could have added anything more to this day if we tried—except for dinner. What are the chances we would dine with another mother/daughter travel duo from southeastern Wisconsin. Must be that "Midwestern Friendly" that drew us to Kathy and her mom Dorita, half way around the world.

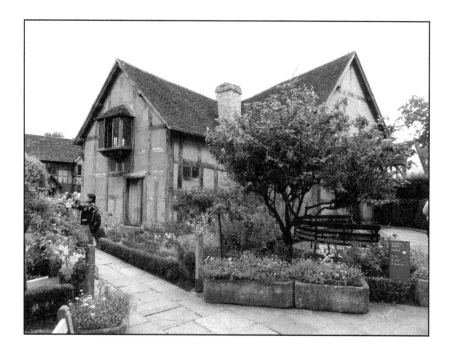

Wales, Bath, and Castle Combe
8-7-14

This day's journey took us 112 miles west through an incredibly scenic English countryside. As we approached the Elizabethan village of Broadway, we marveled at the vistas of the Cotswold Hills. The beautiful homes and the quaint shops were more than charming; I can only imagine what it must have been like to live there.

With barely enough time to take pictures, we continued on to Wales to see the romantic ruins of 12th-century Tintern Abbey. This drive was particularly scenic, with rolling hills, several sheep farms and the River Wye straddled between lush greenery.

Tintern Abbey was founded in 1131 by Cistercian monks who farmed the properties for hundreds of years. It was during the 16th century when Henry VIII led the English Reformation (that was when the Church of England broke away from the authority of the Pope and the Catholic Church) that the Abbey was left to fall into ruin. Now it is considered one of the most romantic ruins in the world, attracting visitors from around the globe.

We were treated to more picturesque countryside as we made our way to the Georgian city of Bath and the amazing excavations of the Roman Baths. The ancient Roman Baths and Temple date back prior to 76 AD. After the Romans left Britain around the 5th century, the baths fell

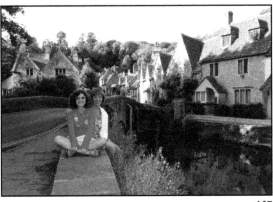

into decay and were eventually covered up. It wasn't until 1880 when sewer workers repairing a leak discovered the ancient baths and its treasures.

One final stop for the night was the picture-book 13th century village of Castle Combe. This town was so lovely, it was voted the prettiest village in the UK. It also was used as a location for the film "Dr. Dolittle," and more recently "War Horse."

We strolled along the river, discovered a 400-year-old door, and had a delightful dinner with British ale at the White Hart Pub (the drinking age in the UK was 18).

Stonehenge, Salisbury, and Brighton 8-8-14

It was a short night's sleep, but a sound one after an incredibly busy day yesterday. I was awakened by my alarm, but also by a flock of seagulls who apparently had been living on the ledge of our hotel room for some time now. After talking with others is our group, it was good to know I wasn't the only one.

I caught a quick nap on our way to Stonehenge, a prehistoric, mysterious circle of upright stones in southern England. Good thing, because I wanted to be wide awake to learn about one of the most famous sites in the world.

Archeologists believe the enormous sarsen (a type of hard sandstone) stones were raised in a horseshoe and a circle 4,500 years ago, with smaller bluestones placed in between them. There were originally 30 upright stones—17 still stand. There is no evidence as to how these 30+ ton stones got there; although they came from an area 19 miles to the north. The bluestones came from the south of Wales, nearly 200 miles away.

It is believed that Stonehenge served as a type of temple with important emphasis placed on the position of the sun. It also served as a burial ground with over 100 burial mounds surrounding the stones.

The first known excavation of Stonehenge was done in the 17th century. By the 20th century, Stonehenge began to be seen as a place of religious significance, and the monument became protected. In 1918 a national restoration of the structure began, and in 1978 direct access to the stones became restricted to prevent vandalism and other damage. Excavations continue; the mystery is still unraveling.

Our next stop brought us to the town of Salisbury, filled with Early English Gothic architecture, and home to the best preserved original Magna Carta, which is inside the Salisbury Cathedral.

Construction of the Salisbury Cathedral began in 1220. It was built in 38 years using 70,000 tons of stone, 2,800 tons of oak, and 420 tons of lead. The spire is Britain's tallest and weighs 6,500 tons!

It also houses the world's oldest working mechanical clock, built in 1386.

The Magna Carta on display in the cathedral's Chapter House is the best preserved of the four originals, dating back to 1215. Written in Latin, with a quill pen on treated animal skin, the charter was forced on King John by barons who were unhappy with the way he was ruling England.

For the protection of this fragile document, no photography is allowed in the room.

Our final stop for that night, was the seaside resort town of Brighton, along the English Channel. A two-hour bus ride turned into nearly three as we got stuck in—wait for it—rush hour traffic!

As we approached the town and pulled up to our hotel, the shoreline—complete with a pier and Ferris wheel—reminded me briefly of our beautiful skyline and Navy Pier.

When we checked in and I saw the view from our room, I knew I was still a continent away, continuing our adventure through historic England.

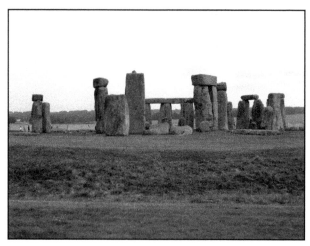

Leeds Castle 8-9-14

All was quiet as we pulled out of Brighton and made our way north toward Kent County—destination, Leeds Castle.

We made a quick stop along the way at the delightful town of Turnbridge Wells, a Georgian village where many of the shops began as residences in the 1600s.

It was time for a quick latte and then off to the magnificent Leeds Castle. Known as "the loveliest castle in the world," there are 1,000 years of history here.

Leeds Castle was originally the site of a manor of the Royal Saxon Family around the 9th century. It was used during the Medieval and Tudor periods by a variety of royalty. In 1519, King Henry VIII transformed the castle for his first wife Catherine of Aragon.

In 1552, Leeds Castle was granted to Sir Anthony St Leger, of Ulcombe near Leeds for a yearly rental of £10 for his services to Henry VIII during the uprising in Ireland. It remained in private ownership for over 400 years.

Since 1974, Leeds Castle Foundation, a private charitable trust, has owned the castle. It is a working castle, kept as a living house, with bedrooms that regularly accommodate guests at weddings, conferences, and banquets. It even hosted the G8 Environment Ministers' Meeting in 1998. With 500 acres of formal gardens and beautiful parkland, Leeds Castle is open

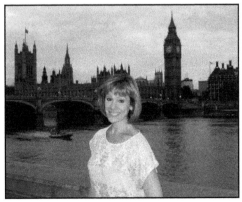

to the public. In the last several decades, over 10 million people have visited the castle.

Make that over 10 million and ONE!

The guided portion of our fabulous adventure ended on a high note as we left Leeds Castle, and made our way back to London. We bade farewell to our delightful guide Niki. Luckily Sara and I then had several days on our own to explore all facets of London.

Inside Buckingham Palace 8-10-14

With the organized tour portion of our British trip behind us, this day's pace was a little less hectic. I had booked a tour inside the State Rooms at Buckingham Palace, which happily for us, was only open between late July and September when the Queen was on holiday. Our hotel was conveniently located just east of the River Thames and two tube stops from the Palace.

We had been so lucky weather-wise, up until today, and of course trying to pack light I did not bring with any rain gear. Fortunately, it was a light drizzle during our walk through Green Park to Buckingham Palace. We arrived early, giving us time to shop before touring the Palace. Not only was I able to get some gifts for friends and family, we were able to purchase a couple small umbrellas to get us through the day, with the "Buckingham Palace" emblem on them no less.

With so many trying to escape the wet weather, the queue to get in was pretty tight. No pictures were allowed inside the palace, same as the White House, but they were allowed outside, so I did snap many pictures from every side of the Palace.

Buckingham Palace is a working Palace, where Her Majesty The Queen carries out her official and ceremonial duties as head of State of the UK and Head of the Commonwealth. The Palace has 775 rooms, including 19 staterooms, 52 royal and guest bedrooms, 188 staff bedrooms, 92 offices and 78 bathrooms! Some 450 people work in the palace. It is furnished with more than 20,000 pieces of art.

Buckingham Palace's garden covers 40 acres. It is home to 30 different species of birds and more than 350 different wild flowers.

After the tour, which included the special exhibit "Royal Childhood"—a display of toys, family gifts and childhood outfits of the royal children—Sara and I had lunch at the Garden Café on the Palace's West Terrace.

Since the rain had stopped, traffic was light, and a bike-a-thon was just finishing, we decided to walk back.

Walking is always better than driving/commuting, because you can see so much more—like a clothing shop unique to the UK. (Yes, I bought her the dress!)

By the time we left the store, it had started raining again, so walking around Piccadilly Circus didn't seem so appealing. At least we had those umbrellas now!

We opted for a tube ride back to the hotel, had light snacks for dinner, watched a movie and made a chill night of it.

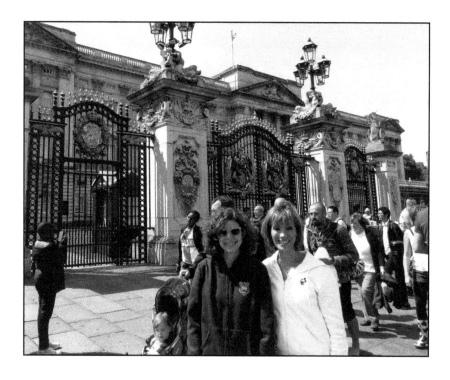

Up The Shard 8-11-14

Our morning started with a quick trip on the Tube to London's newest landmark, The Shard (think Willis Tower). This modern marvel opened in February of 2013 and at the time was Europe's tallest building.

Seventy-two stories high, it houses the Shangri-La Hotel, exclusive residences, restaurants, businesses, and viewing galleries on the 68, 69 and 72 floors that give a spectacular 360-degree view for up to 40 miles! To the south, one can see the London Eye (Ferris wheel), Buckingham Palace, Parliament, and Big Ben.

To the west, there's an amazing view of the River Thames and several bridges that cross it, including the Waterloo, Blackfriars and Millennium.

The north view features London Bridge, Tower 42, Broadgate Tower, Lloyds of London and Gherkin.

The east view—my favorite—highlighted the magnificent Tower Bridge, The Tower of London, City Hall, and off in the distance, the Olympic Stadium.

The Shard is 1,016 feet high, has 44 lifts (elevators) that travel up to 6 meters per second, and its construction consists of 11,000 glass panels!

After admiring the view for a couple hours, we decided to go back and walk around Piccadilly Circus and Trafalgar Square sans the rain. The sun was shining at Piccadilly Circus. As we walked among the historic buildings, Sara wanted to know why this area was called "Piccadilly Circus" when it clearly was NOT a circus!

Piccadilly Circus was built in 1819 in order to connect Regent Street and Piccadilly Street. The word 'Circus' for 'circle' refers to the round-about around which the traffic circulated. Very "Readers Digest" explanation.

We stopped for a quick bite to eat, and began making our way to Trafalgar Square. As soon as we arrived, so did the rain! Good thing the National Gallery was right there—made for a very interesting and culturally educational shelter.

So much art, so little time. We made our way back to the tube, heading to our hotel to get ready for dinner and theatre in London's famous West End. Don't forget—MIND THE GAP!

We had dinner at The Globe, a local pub perfect for fish n' chips and a lager. Then on to the Theatre Royal Drury Lane to see "Charlie and The Chocolate Factory."

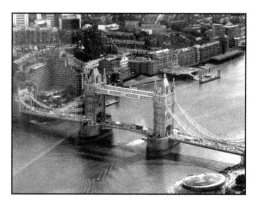

This mouth-watering musical was so good; it had us craving chocolate by intermission. After the show, Sara was lucky enough to get a couple of autographs from the child stars who played Charlie and Augustus.

"...There is no life I know to compare with pure imagination, living there you'll be free, if you truly wish to be..."

Abbey Road 8-13-14

I felt like our London adventure had come full circle. The first day we arrived, my friend Fred gave us a quick tour of the St. John's Wood district and the famous Abbey Road site and studio. As we approached our last days in London, the "In My Life" Beatles tour brought us back to the same spot!

Outside the Marylebone Station, we met up with Richard Porter, one of the best walking tour guides in London, and an expert on all things Beatles. Our first stop was right next to the station where they filmed the opening scenes for "A Hard Day's Night."

Next stop, the registry office where two of the Beatles were married, Paul and Linda McCartney, and Ringo Starr and Barbara Bach.

We took a short walk to #34 Montagu, a building with a lot of Beatles history. Ringo lived there; his first son Zach (a drummer with The Who) was born at that time. Paul wrote "Eleanor Rigby" there. And it's the building where the infamous John and Yoko "Two Virgins" picture was taken.

On to Baker Street. The Marsh & Parsons building is the former Apple Shop, which had the psychedelic mural painted on the wall.

Our next stop was at 57 Wimpole Street, the home of Dr. Richard Asher and his wife Margaret. Paul dated their daughter, actress Jane Asher, during the early years and spent much time there. It's where Lennon and McCartney wrote "I Want To Hold Your Hand."

Saving the best for last, we wrapped up our tour in front of the legendary Abbey Road Studios and site of the iconic album cover. Ninety percent of the Beatles' music was recorded at that studio. By the way, the album was NOT named after the studio, but the road where the studio is located. Back then, the studio was called EMI; it didn't become Abbey Road Studios until after the album came out.

Our guide Richard shared many stories at this site; how the original title of the "Abbey Road" album was to be called "Everest" and the cover photo to be shot at Mt. Everest. They decided upon Abbey Road as a closer and warmer site. There were many tales of fans, who would gather outside the studio in hopes of meeting their musical idols. Two lucky fans got that and more in 1968, when the Beatles were recording "Across The Universe."

We couldn't leave without the traditional signing of the wall in front of the studio, and one more shot at taking a picture along the crosswalk.

We got our share of Beatles souvenirs at The Beatles Coffee Shop, outside the St. John's Wood Station, including an autographed copy of Richard's book.

A great day—in my life!

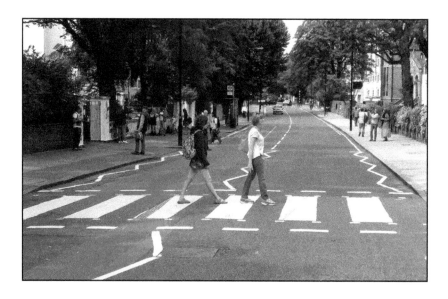

Back Home 8-15-14

It is said, all good things must come to an end, and such was the case with our magnificent British adventure. I wanted to wrap things up with an easy, fun day and just soak up everything we had experienced this side of the pond. I chose two of our favorite things: shopping and theatre. At this point, we had become totally acclimated to the Tube, which I might add is the most efficient, user-friendly, clean and safe public transportation system I had ever experienced.

Covent Garden is right next to the theatre district; it's filled with everything from quaint shops and boutiques to familiar big-name retailers. This venture was all about the shoes!

Good thing the Noel Coward Theatre was willing to hold our bags in coat check, while we caught the matinee of the new hit comedy, "Shakespeare In Love." Adapted from the Oscar-winning film, this play was outstanding. Once again, we waited patiently at the stage door to see which actors might appear to sign playbills and take pictures. We were star-struck.

After getting our fill of celebrity moments, I just wanted to walk around Covent Garden and take it all in—the sights, the sounds, the people—memories to last a lifetime.

One last Tube ride back to Waterloo Station and it was time to pack up and get ready to head home.

Our flight home was without incident—other

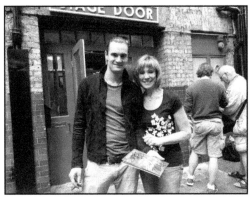

than the eight-hour duration, and a couple vocal infants! After an experience in world history unlike any found in a text book. We arrived back home refreshed, revitalized and with a new appreciation of our mates overseas.

Life

A Happy Ending 9-7-14

This is the story of "Sleep Baby," a story that I feared would have a terrible outcome! Sleep Baby was my daughter's security doll, so to speak. A small, plush, stuffed baby doll that she had slept with since infancy. It had been mended, stitched and re-stuffed more times than I could remember. It had traveled the world—from summer camp and school trips to family vacations in the U.S. and abroad. Yes, Sleep Baby had led a good life—until our latest trip overseas.

When Sara and I took our amazing vacation to the UK, Sleep Baby was right along side for the eight-hour flight from O'Hare to Heathrow.

The first half of our trip was an organized tour of southern England, which meant staying at a different hotel in a different city almost every night. Each morning before we'd check out, we'd both do the "sweep" to make sure we didn't leave anything behind.

I'm sure by now you know where I'm heading with this. An hour after we left our hotel in Bath, England, on the bus to visit Stonehenge, Sara realized to her horror she had left Sleep Baby in our room at the Hilton Bath City Hotel! I immediately went into action, frantically searching for the hotel phone number. Of course it was impossible to get through, which only heightened my anxiety and Sara's tears. Our tour guide Niki assured me that while we toured Stonehenge, she would get in touch with the hotel to see if housekeeping had retrieved the beloved doll.

Miraculously, Niki did get in touch with the hotel, and they did find Sleep Baby! Since we were headed to London for the next five days, I suggested she have them mail the doll to our London hotel so we could reunite Sara and Sleep Baby before we returned home. Surely it would arrive within six days. Wrong.

Every day in London we checked with the concierge, anxiously awaiting Sleep Baby's arrival, but with no luck. The day before we were to check out I called the Hilton Bath City Hotel to see if they could track it down. They said the doll was in transit and should arrive before we had to leave. Obviously, that didn't happen. At this point, Sara, who was just weeks from heading off to college, said to me, "It's okay Mom. I knew I'd have to give it up sometime." Call me sentimental, call me crazy, call me heartbroken—I wasn't giving up!

The day after we returned to Chicago, I called the Hilton Bath City Hotel one more time with the ongoing saga of Sleep Baby, and received a very sympathetic ear from manager Joanne Blakey, who knew the importance of the aforementioned doll. She promised to track it down once it arrived in London, have it sent BACK to the Hilton Bath City Hotel, where she would take responsibility to have it mailed back to us in the states.

Yes, this story does have a happy ending. I tracked that silly doll's voyage for weeks through the Royal Mail Parcelforce, and finally, the Friday before Labor Day, I received notification that a package was waiting for me at the Oak Park Post Office. Joanne, I can't thank you enough for this incredible act of kindness!

Sara returned to her dorm after the long holiday weekend with Sleep Baby by her side. While Sara may not "need" the security of her childhood doll as she makes the transition into college, at least she can make the decision to move on without it on her terms.

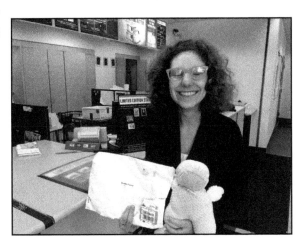

Ten Years of Happily Ever After
6-2-15

Marriage isn't easy—admittedly who among us doesn't wish the romance stage would last forever. In reality, it takes a lot of work, compromise, and sacrifice to make a marriage last. But when you find the right person, it's worth the blood sweat and tears to hold true to those vows.

On June 11, 2015 Glenn and I celebrated our 10th wedding anniversary. It was a fairy tale wedding, "Made in Chicago," at the Walnut Room at Marshall Fields! I felt like Cinderella, with my handsome prince. At the time, I had no idea what the future had in store for me, and frankly, I didn't care.

Shortly after our 1st anniversary I was diagnosed with Stage 4 Breast Cancer. Glenn stood by me every step of the way, accompanying me to every oncologist appointment; he still does to this day.

He helped raise Sara as his own, merging seamlessly into our kooky blended family of half-siblings and step-siblings. That being said, it wasn't always smooth sailing—there were plenty of rough patches, and some hurdles that seemed awfully steep at the time. But I made a vow, for better or worse, and the optimist in me always prevails!

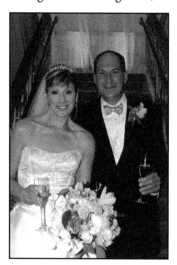

So here we were, at the time 10 years down the road, and Glenn and I were heading to Hawaii to renew our vows. My daughter and my parents were joining us for a sunset ceremony the following week that took place along the beach in Maui— the same place where we honeymooned 10 years ago!

Travel: Hawaii

Honolulu 6-10-15

When my husband and I first traveled to Hawaii, we were newly-weds, honeymooning in a tropical paradise.

Ten years later, we had returned to renew our vows, this time bringing my daughter and my parents to share in our celebration.

The first half of the trip was under our belt—3 days in O'ahu for some sun, sand, and sightseeing. We did a little shopping at Hilo Hattie's; the world was our oyster, at The Pearl Factory, and we savored a breathtaking sunset over the Pacific Ocean.

The next day was particularly poignant, as we visited Pearl Harbor, a first for my Dad, who is retired Air Force/Air National Guard.

Our tour started with a moving documentary that included historic footage of the Japanese attack on the U.S Naval Base at Pearl Harbor, December 7, 1941, which propelled America into World War II. There were two exhibit galleries, explaining events that lead up to the war, and the actual attack.

A Navy shuttle boat took visitors to the USS Arizona Memorial, which was built over the sunken hull of the battleship.

It honors the 1,177 crewmen who died on that "date which will live in infamy." It was a heartbreaking, but most beautiful tribute. A humbling experience, indeed.

Our evening ended with another incredible sunset, and a re-creation of a picture we took on our honeymoon along Waikiki Beach with Diamond Head as our backdrop.

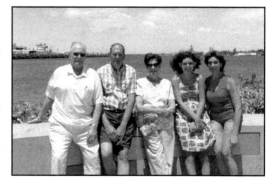

Maui 6-12-15

Maui was magical; its beauty was beyond words. Each incredible sunrise, every picturesque sunset–it was only fitting to renew our 10th anniversary wedding vows in this tropical paradise. We were blessed to have my parents, daughter, and dear friend Julie, join us on this special day.

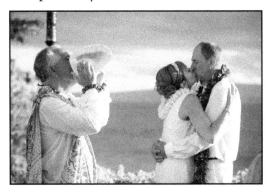

After a magnificent celebration, we had two days to explore the island. Having driven the road to Hana on our honeymoon 10 years ago, we opted to drive to the summit of Haleakala this time around. It was 90 minutes of twists and turns through the mountains of this dormant volcano up to an altitude of 10,000 feet!

We were lucky; clear skies welcomed us as we reached the top. The view was spectacular! Nothing could prepare you for the deeply sculpted, richly colored landscape.

It reminded me of the Painted Desert. Mostly barren, there was some plant life speckled through the cinder rock, including a rare species only found on Haleakala.

As we ventured onto our final day in Maui, and after another twisty-turn drive down the mountain, we were treated to yet another spectacular sunset.

We decided to end the week by snorkeling at two very different beaches. We began at Ahihi Kinau Natural Area Reserve. Because it was a marine life conservation district, no fishing was allowed, making it an amazing place to snorkel.

We left the lava rock coast of Ahihi Bay went to the sandy shores of Ulua-Mokapu Beach which was one of southern Maui's most popular snorkel beaches. It was with with good reason–the coastline was a favorite hang-out of the magnificent Hawaiian Sea Turtles.

One last dinner with my fabulous family included one final Hawaiian sunset and one more sunrise along the beach before we headed back to Chicago with a lifetime of magnificent memories.

Travel: Walt Disney World

Reliving The Magic 9-7-15

My first magical encounter with Mickey & Co. was at a time when the "Happiest Place On Earth" was still undeveloped swampland in central Florida. I was 10, and could barely contain my excitement at our first big family trip to Disneyland in Anaheim, California. I was born during the Mouseketeers era, grew up watching "The Wonderful World of Disney" and now I was about to get my own set of ears!

The Magic Kingdom was the most magical place I'd ever seen, so it was a no-brainer I would want to share this experience with my own daughter. Sara's first encounter with Mickey & Co. was on a family vacation to southern California, which of course included a trip to Disneyland. Sara was barely two—she doesn't remember it at all.

We tried again two years later with a weeklong family trip to Walt Disney World in Florida. I have great memories of that trip—seeing the thrill and excitement of Disney through her eyes. Sara, on the other hand, remembered nothing.

The next year I planned a Mother/Daughter trip to Walt Disney World (WDW) during spring break. This trip has VERY vivid memories for both of us, but not what you'd expect from the "Happiest Place On Earth."

Sara and I were having dinner at the Liberty Tree Tavern in the Magic Kingdom. Crowds were gathering outside the restaurant, waiting for the Main Street Electrical Parade. Sara, being a typical four-year-old was making a mess with coloring paper and asked if she could throw it out. Seeing a garbage can around the corner, I agreed, since I felt I could keep my eye on her.

BIG mistake—she darted around the corner and when she didn't come right back, I went to look for her. She was nowhere in sight! With crowds thickening for the oncoming parade, panic set in, especially since the doors to the restaurant were open.

My eyes wide with fear, I found a manager, told her my little girl was missing, gave them a description, and prayed for her return. Within minutes that seemed like an eternity, my precious baby casually walked back to the table, wondering what all the fuss was about. Sara remembers this event VERY clearly!

This is what she has explained about the incident, "I was shredding paper and stuffing it in my pocket and wanted to get rid of it. I asked you if I could go around the corner to throw out the paper because it was bothering me. You said, yes, so I went around the corner but couldn't find the garbage. I went into the bathroom because I figured I'd find one there. Once I got to the bathroom, I thought I should go, so I waited in line. Then I went back to the table, not thinking anything was wrong. When I saw you all freaked out, I freaked out and we were both crying! But then Goofy came over and calmed us down. We finished our dinner and watched the parade like every other normal family."

The other strong memory I have that Sara doesn't remember is a fun one. On Cinderella's Carousel, she would only ride the horse with the roses. Forgive me for giving in to this, but we waited in line, letting others go ahead, so she would be first and be able to get on that particular darned horse. On subsequent trips, I never let her forget this.

Our next Disney adventure was 2005, the summer I remarried; Sara was 10. We have selective memories here—mine are of a new blended family, enjoying the rides, attractions and characters at this magical theme park. Sara remembers The Lego Store at Downtown Disney, waiting in a LONG line for Splash Mountain and deciding at the last minute she was too scared to ride it. She also recalled the queasy feeling my husband and stepson had after riding Mission Space at EPCOT. Needless to say, Sara and I did NOT go on that ride!

Our memories started to gel during the next family trip to WDW. Thirteen-year-old Sara was more than willing to ride Space Mountain with me, several times. We got caught up in the pin collection craze, and couldn't get enough of the wave pool at Typhoon Lagoon. We wisely did not partake in "Humunga Kowabunga" and risk a bathing suit wedgie.

We officially made Sara a Disney Princess by celebrating her Sweet 16 at Disney World. I took her and two of her "besties" for a long birthday weekend; I don't know who had more fun!

The true test would be a surprise "Destination Disney" for her 18th birthday with 10 family members. Could I pull it off? I told her to pack for fun-in-the-sun. As soon as we got to the airport, she knew exactly where we were going. But when she saw the rest of the family at the hotel, she was speechless. Mission accomplished.

Before Sara returned to college, I made the decision to take another mother/daughter WDW trip. Doing Disney with the almost 20-year-old Sara was a much different, yet incredibly fulfilling experience. She was a great travel buddy; we enjoyed the same things and liked to make the most of our time, without ending up on the brink of exhaustion.

As I relive these magical vacations, I have a greater appreciation for the family trips of my youth, and the special times spent with my mom. I also understand all too well the emptiness my mother felt as I spread my wings into young adulthood.

As for Sara, regardless of age, she will always be my Disney Princess.

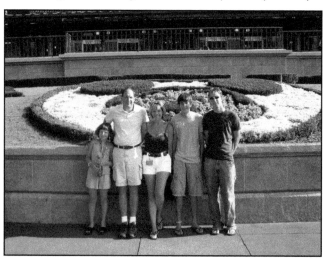

Some of Disney's Hidden Magic
11-22-15

Spoiler Alert—if you don't want to know some of the hidden ways Disney's Magic Kingdom works, stop now. On the other hand, if you love behind-the-scenes stories, read on my friend.

Mind you, any time we went behind the scenes, or into the famed "Utilidors," no picture taking was allowed. Being a "Cast Member" myself (ABC is owned by Disney), I was respectful of that rule. The rest—fair game. So here goes.

Let's start with the park entrance—Disney designed it like a theatre. The ticket area is the "lobby," the tunnels under the train station are lined with "coming attraction" posters—the train station itself is the curtain, and once you go through it and enter the Magic Kingdom, the walkway is red, as you walk the "red carpet."

The buildings on Main Street were built with "forced perspective" to make the street look longer than it is. The first floor in most multi-story buildings on Main Street was regular size, but the second and third floors were built at a smaller scale giving the illusion that the buildings were taller than they actually were.

Same concept with Cinderella's Castle—the bricks got smaller the higher up the castle went. Main Street sloped upward, approaching the castle, making it easier for tired visitors to walk down hill at the end of their day. (It was so subtle; the park visitors didn't notice this strategy.)

Fun Fact—None of the American flags flying high above Main Street had 50 stars. The reason, flags with less than 50 stars don't count as real flags, and therefore don't have to be taken down in bad weather or lit at night. The only true flag, full of 50 stars, waved over Town Square in the front of the park.

Moving on to Liberty Square. The Liberty Bell replica was cast from the mold of the actual Liberty Bell. The crack in the bell, however, had to be recreated.

163

Fun facts at the Haunted Mansion—It's the only attraction that is included in every Magic Kingdom Theme Park in the world, but is located within a different land in each park.

Up or down? The famous stretching room, where you first enter the attraction, descends at Disneyland, but at Walt Disney World the ceiling rises while guests stayed on the same level.

The Narrator in the Haunted Mansion was the late voice actor, Paul Frees. His voice was used in many other WDW attractions, including the Hall of Presidents and Pirates of the Caribbean. Frees was also the voice of Boris Badenov (from the Rocky and Bullwinkle Show) and The Pillsbury Doughboy.

What about the famed "Utilidors?" Short for Utility Corridors, this backstage area is used for park operations, out of guests' sight, to keep the magic intact.

Fun fact—Do to the high water table, the Utilidor tunnels were built before the theme park at ground level. The Magic Kingdom was built above ground level on the second, and in some cases, third story. The incline was so gradual, we didn't even notice it as we walked through the park.

You would never see a garbage truck in the parks. That's because Disney uses an AVAC (Automated Vacuum-Assisted Collection) system instead. Giant air pressurized tubes jet trash to a processing area behind Splash Mountain—at over 60 MPH. It's all concealed within the Utilidors.

Here's another behind-the-scenes tidbit. Disney animators and theme park "imagineers" have been incorporating "hidden Mickeys" (the three circles that form the iconic Mickey silhouette) for decades; first in animated films, then carried over into the theme parks.

It started as an inside joke that is now a popular pastime for park guests—in fact, one employee told me in the early days, animators were not allowed to take credit for their drawings, so incorporating a "hidden Mickey" in a spot only they knew, was their way of putting a signature on their work.

For those of you wondering about those odd mouse ears that Sara wore throughout the trip, they were actually rabbit ears. Oswald The

Lucky Rabbit was Walt Disney's first cartoon creation in 1927. Walt lost the character to his distributors in 1928, because unbeknown to Disney, the distributors contractually owned the rights to Oswald. Of course, that's when Mickey Mouse was born in Oswald's place, and the rest, as they say, is history.

Fun fact—The Disney Company was able to regain the rights to Oswald in 2006 in a unique trade deal. With all the media mergers over the years, Disney/ABC/ESPN traded sportscaster Al Michaels to NBC/Universal for the rights to Oswald along with 26 vintage Oswald cartoons.

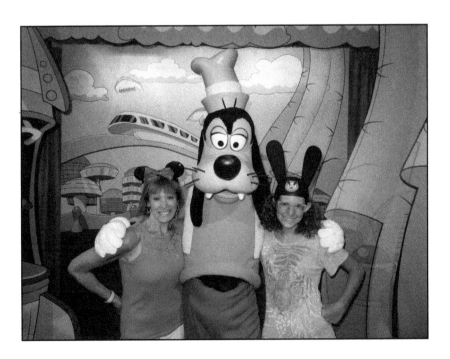

Travel: New Orleans

The French Quarter 3-18-16

Iam most fortunate that my daughter chooses to spend spring break traveling with me, rather than with her besties. On the other hand, I always have taken her on some amazing adventures—this time to the Big Easy.

The last time Sara and I were in New Orleans was as part of a tour. We only spent a few days there—not nearly enough to experience all that NOLA had to offer. We sampled many types of food (Sara got hooked on Shrimp & Grits) and we listened to fabulous jazz music.

This time we would be there for one week, enough time to explore much of what this incredible city had to offer.

Our first day in the Big Easy was anything but. Rain and cool temperatures greeted us, making it a little challenging to walk through the French Quarter—but the sights, sounds and flavors of New Orleans beckoned—and we answered the call.

Sara thoroughly enjoyed her first Muffaletta at Cafe Maspero (very little convincing on my part). We took shelter from the wind and rain in the French Market, marveled at the unique items, and acted like total tourists.

There's no doubt, New Orleans is a GREAT place to people watch, but when it comes to music, words can't begin to describe it.

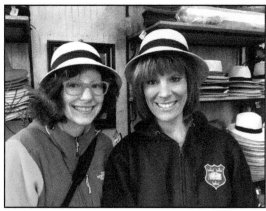

The National World War II Museum 3-20-16

This day's adventure took us out of the French Quarter and back in time. In order to take in more sights and sounds of The Crescent City, we decided to take the 25-minute walk to the National World War II Museum.

Our visit to the National World War II Museum was quite a powerful experience. This collection of artifacts, interactive exhibits, and moving personal accounts explained the war in a way that informs, educates and inspires.

Because my dad, Master Sergeant Jack Varon, is retired Air Force and Air National Guard, both Sara and I took a special interest in the Boeing Center exhibit.

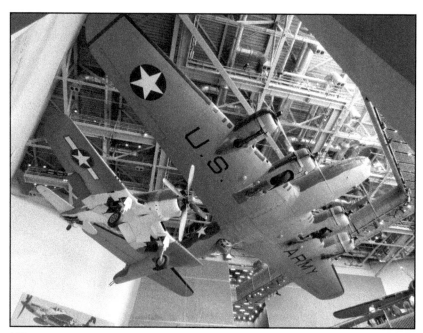

The Sights and Sounds of NOLA
3-22-16

The clear, blue sky gave way to brilliant sunlight cast over the French Quarter, making it a perfect day to walk through historic Jackson Square, capturing images along the way.

We had to start our day the NOLA way, with a tasty beignet. Here was where the beauty of social media really kicked in—as suggested by Facebook fans, rather than stand in a LONG line at Cafe Du Monde, we went across the street to New Orleans Famous Beignets & Coffee, which were just as delicious.

Taking another cue from Facebook fans, we took the short walk to Mr. B's Bistro for their famous BBQ shrimp—a messy, but delicious experience.

The biggest draw for me continued to be the music, pure and simple. From blues to jazz and everything in between, it drew me in; I became immersed in the rhythms of this magical city.

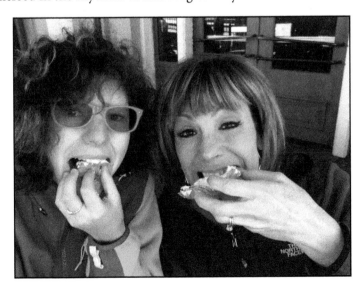

Haunted New Orleans 3-23-16

Our day was filled with history, hauntings, fact and myth. Regardless of what you believe, it was interesting. We started with the New Orleans History Walking Tour of St. Louis Cemetery, the oldest in the Crescent City. Although we walked along the block where the first cemetery, St. Peter, was located in the 1700's, it no longer exists. We were told that remains had recently been found during construction in the area.

Our tour guide showed us the variety of above ground tombs from the oldest gravesite to long wall vaults, family tombs and society tombs.

St. Louis Cemetery's most famous grave site is that of Voodoo priestess Marie Laveau. It is customary to make a wish on her tomb. (We did!)

Our next adventure took us uptown for the Haunted Garden District Walking Tour. We started at—you guessed it—another cemetery! Lafayette Cemetery was built in the mid-1800s on the site of a former plantation. Scenes from "Double Jeopardy" and "Interview With A Vampire" were shot here.

The haunted stories were a bit creepy—in 1847 nearly 3,000 people died of yellow fever. More than 600 are buried at Lafayette. As our tour guide explained, some were mistakenly buried alive! Sounds of screams and moans had been reported coming from the tombs. Upon inspection, scratch marks and finger nail residue reportedly were found inside the tombs!

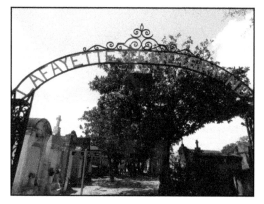

Our tour continued through the upscale Garden District, with its historic mansions and haunted homes. Sandra Bullock has a residence here (not haunted) and author Anne Rice ("The Vampire Chronicles") owned a home here (very haunted!).

Two tours in one day were more than enough. We rode the historic trolley back toward the French Quarter, picking up a little street history along the way.

The Bayou 3-23-16

I was somewhat hesitant, but my daughter didn't blink an eye. So off we went, on a kayak tour down the bayou. We took the Lake Pontchartrain Causeway—the world's longest bridge over a body of water (almost 24 miles) to Fontainebleau State Park, a 2,800-acre park along the shores of Lake Pontchartrain.

There were 10 in our group, some novices, some experienced, all hoping to see alligators. We saw a variety of plant life through the swamps and marsh, from tall cypress trees to lacy Spanish moss.

And about those wildlife sightings? Well, you can see for yourself.

A special thanks to our tour guide Matt and all the folks at Canoe & Trail Adventures for making this experience so memorable.

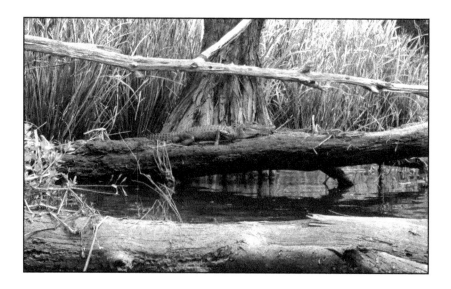

Travel: New England and Canada

Philadelphia 8-7-16

Let me state for the record, this was going to be the most ambitious road trip we had ever taken to date. Glenn, Sara, and I would be driving through eight states in the New England area and two Canadian provinces in 12 days. We chose this route because these are beautiful and historic places we had never seen...and we LOVE adventure!

Our road trip began in Philadelphia, a city with more history than I could ever explain. It was our nation's first capital from 1790 to 1800. The city of "brotherly love" was named by Quaker William Penn in the late 1600s, derived from the Greek words "phileo" (to love) and "adelphos" (brother).

We got a quick lay of the land at Independence Park, home of several sites associated with the American Revolution and our nation's founding history. We stood on the site of the home and executive offices of our first two presidents—George Washington from 1790 to 1797 and John Adams from 1797 to 1800.

We saw a very powerful exhibit and theatrical presentation at The National Constitution Center, which dug deep into the history of "We, the people..."

It was much quieter after the Democratic National Convention, but the event definitely left its mark. Fifty-seven fiberglass "Donkeys Around Town" (think 'Cows on Parade') representing participating convention delegations

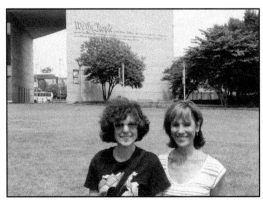

were on display. And of course, more political paraphernalia than you could imagine.

We stopped by the U.S. mint, but couldn't make a withdrawal (they were closed!).

As if we didn't have enough to see and do, we also squeezed in some family time, visiting cousins in Baltimore, then back to sightseeing in Philly. Like I said, a very ambitious schedule indeed!

Independence Hall 8-8-16

There is an overwhelming sense of patriotism that takes hold when you explore Independence National Historical Park in Philadelphia. This is where the United States was born—where the Declaration of Independence was created and the Constitution was signed. We began our day with the most recognized symbol of America's quest for freedom, the Liberty Bell

The 2,080-pound State House bell was hung in the Pennsylvania State House (now Independence Hall) in 1753 to summon the State Assembly to work. It wasn't until the 1830's that abolitionists wishing to end slavery named it the Liberty Bell. The infamous crack happened around 1846—no one knows exactly how or why, but the message of freedom still rings out loud and clear.

Our next stop, Independence Hall. This was originally the Pennsylvania State House, but from 1790 to 1800 it served as the U.S. Supreme Court, the U.S. Congress and the Assembly Room where the Declaration of Independence and the Constitution were created.

Trying to squeeze as much into one day as possible, we walked north on 5th Street to the U.S. Mint for a self-guided tour to see how coins are made. These coins are pressed so fast—12 per second, 750 each minute. So far that year more than 6 billion coins had been made at this facility. There were no pictures allowed in the coin press area, but nobody said anything about the gift shop!

All this walking/touring gave us quite an appetite. We decided to check out Reading Terminal Market for lunch. With over 75 vendors, and every ethnic food you could imagine, the choices were overwhelming—but what a way to calm those hunger pangs.

We still had a couple hours until closing time for most historic sites, so tummies full, we forged ahead. The Declaration house (rebuilt in

1975) is where Thomas Jefferson, in June of 1776, drafted the Declaration of Independence.

There was so much Benjamin Franklin history there, we had to take in Franklin Court and the Market St. houses. Benjamin Franklin owned a large house in the courtyard behind several homes on Market Street. Today, you can only see a "ghost house" or frame of where his home stood, as well as a lower level kitchen floor that was discovered and protected.

On our last stop were the oldest homes I had ever seen on American soil. Elfreth's Alley is known as "Our nation's oldest residential street" dating back to 1702. There are over 30 homes on this narrow stretch of road, most still occupied.

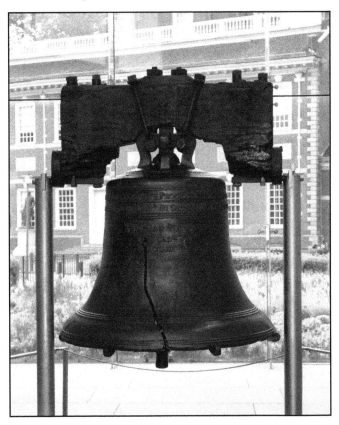

NYC 8-9-16

There's a certain vibe about New York City. The energy surrounds you, encompasses you and welcomes you!

The crowds, the noise, and the construction, even the garbage in the streets—it doesn't matter—the charm of the Big Apple always beckons when I'm out east. Since we were only staying one night, and because of its proximity to both the interstate and Times Square, we decided to try a new "boutique hotel" called the Yotel Hotel...interesting experience.

A quick spot of shopping, a lovely dinner at Rosie O'Grady's on 7th Avenue and a fantastic time at the Tony-nominated musical "School Of Rock" at the Winter Garden Theatre with my fabulous Uncle Malcolm Varon made our visit complete!

We did love NYC, but we were back on the road in the morning, heading to Connecticut.

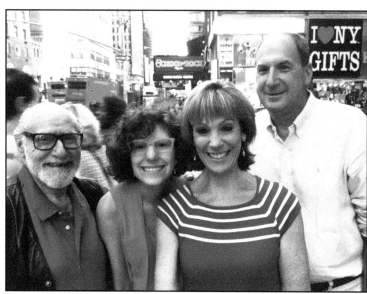

Hartford, CT 8-10-16

So many states, so little time! We decided to make Hartford Connecticut a day stop, spending a few hours exploring the house that Mark Twain, from 1874 to 1891, called home.

Samuel Clemens, aka Mark Twain completed seven books while living in the Hartford home, including *The Adventures of Tom Sawyer* (1876), *A Connecticut Yankee in King Arthur's Court* (1889) and *Adventures of Huckleberry Finn* (1884).

Sam Clemens, his wife Olivia (Livy) and their three children Susy, Clara, and Jean lived in the home. Their first child, a son Langford, died at age two, before the house was built.

There are authentic Clemens items in every room in the house. The Clemens believed it was healthier to sleep sitting up. The pillows were placed at the foot of the bed, as they enjoyed looking at the ornate headboard they purchased in Venice.

The Clemens loved to entertain—12 to 14 guests three times a week, they were among the first to have a telephone wired into their home.

As you might imagine, I really wanted to spend more time at the Mark Twain House & Museum. A huge THANK YOU to the gracious staff, for allowing me to take photos after our tour.

As we continued east, we arrived at our next destination, Yarmouth Port Cape Cod, just in time for

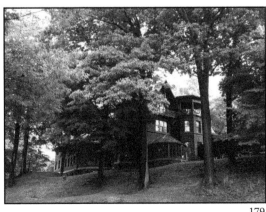

dinner. We were staying at The Inn at Cape Cod; a historic B & B built in 1820. It was every bit as charming as I had anticipated.

We didn't have to go far for a most incredible dinner. The Old Yarmouth Inn, claiming to be the oldest in Cape Cod established in 1696, was right next door. It is listed on the National Register of Historic Places, and our dinner was as impressive, if not more so than the history. Sara and I shared a two-pound lobster, which was stuffed with shrimp and scallops.

Cape Cod 8-12-16

Hard to believe, with all the traveling I've done, I had never stayed at a Bed & Breakfast until this trip. Before becoming a stagecoach hotel in 1830, in 1820, The Inn at Cape Cod was built as a private mansion. It is now listed on the National Register of Historic Places.

Our hosts, Mike and Helen Cassels, were just as charming and welcoming as the inn itself.

We spent the day in Hyannis—with its mid-cape location surrounded by restaurants, B&B's, shopping, island ferries and beaches—it is considered to be the hub of Cape Cod. It is also home to the John F. Kennedy Hyannis Museum and Kennedy Compound. (No, we did not visit; invite must have gotten lost in the mail.) We drove through historic Main Street; along the way we admired the lovely Colonial-style homes.

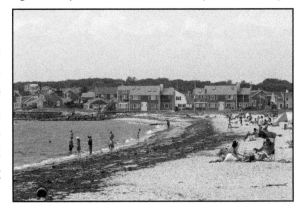

On our abbreviated schedule we wanted to make sure we hit the beach. Kalmus Park Beach was close, breezy, and had a huge parking lot. Bingo!

Boston 8-13-16

A Bostonian told us, "The beauty of New England is its variety—you drive 45 minutes and the scenery is completely different." And so it was as we left the charm and peacefulness of Cape Cod and entered the historic, yet urban streets of Boston.

Our main goal during our one day stay was to walk the Freedom Trail—a 2 and one half mile marked path through downtown Boston that passes 16 sites which are significant to the American Revolutionary story.

We started at Boston Common, American's oldest park, dating back to the 1630s.

Tucked behind the garden was the Massachusetts State House, completed in 1798. The golden dome was once made of wood, and later overlaid with copper by Paul Revere. It was covered with 23-karat gold leaf in 1874. One of the oldest buildings in Beacon Hill, it is the current government building in the state capital.

Across from the State House is Granary Burying Ground, which is the final resting place of many notable Revolutionary heroes, including Paul Revere, Samuel Adams and John Hancock, as well as Benjamin Franklin's parents.

Although there are 2,345 markers, it is estimated that at least 5,000 people were buried there. Since headstones were expensive, it was common to put several members of one family under one headstone with only one name on it.

We passed by the Old South Meeting House where thousands of angry colonists gathered in 1773 to protest a tax and started a revolution with the Boston Tea Party.

We toured the Old State House, which was built in 1713. Decades later, in 1776, the Declaration of Independence was first read from the building's balcony to the people of Boston.

Right behind the Old State House was the site of the Boston Massacre, March 5, 1770.

We continued north to Faneuil Hall, which was built in 1741 as one of America's first public meeting venues and considered "the home of free speech."

Next door was the historic Quincy Market, constructed in 1824. It was designated a National Historic Landmark as one of the nation's largest market complexes. We opted to go there to get some relief from the 90+ degree heat.

We decided to make the Paul Revere House our last stop on the Freedom Trail—one, because it was starting to rain, and two, we were running out of time.

Built around 1680, it's the oldest structure in downtown Boston and the only home on the Freedom Trail.

Based on many recommendations, we stopped for a quick snack on Hanover Street, Boston's "Little Italy," for a mouth-watering cannoli at Mike's Pastry.

On our walk back to the hotel, we passed by the lively Farmer's Market, where vendors were trying to sell off the last of their produce before closing.

Our dinner was at the legendary Legal Seafood— how fabulous to have New England Clam Chowder in New England.

We capped off our evening doing the tourist thing— a stop at the infamous Cheers Bar.

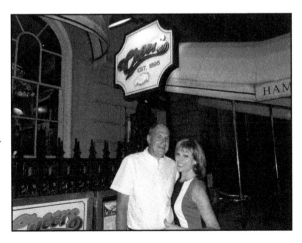

Maine 8-14-16

O ur first day in Maine brought quite the change of scenery. Lush forests filled with tall pines graced each side of the road as we drove through the rolling hills toward Portland.

Portland was the halfway point to Acadia National Park and gave us a great opportunity to see Maine's oldest lighthouse.

Portland Head Lighthouse was first lit in 1791. Construction began several years earlier under the directive of George Washington, while Maine was still part of the state of Massachusetts. It sits along the rocky shores of Cape Elizabeth in Fort Williams Park, and in 1973, was added to the National Register of Historic Places.

As lovely as the cape was, we still had another three-hour drive to Acadia, so off we went. We drove through clouds and light rain, but the scenery was still beautiful and serene.

We arrived at our hotel in time for dinner, but no time to explore Acadia. We opted to go into the charming sea town of Bar Harbor for dinner and shopping — good call. Fresh lobster and a mouth-watering Wild Maine Blueberry Crisp for dessert!

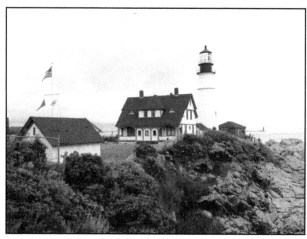

Acadia National Park 8-14-16

It's a good thing we didn't try to watch the sunrise from Cadillac Mountain at Acadia National Park or we would have been sorely disappointed. A thick fog greeted us as we hit the road at 7:00 a.m.

Nonetheless, the park was incredibly beautiful and barely populated at that early morning hour, allowing us free reign to gather some incredible pictures.

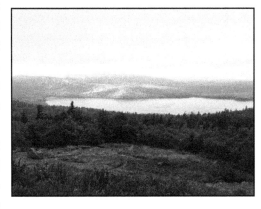

We marveled at Thunder Hole, so named because of the thunderous sound that was made when just the right sized wave rolled into the naturally formed inlet.

We continued along the Park Loop Road to Otter Cliff, one of the highest Atlantic coastal headlands north of Rio de Janeiro. Unfortunately, the fog prevented us from capturing the full view.

As we looped around north toward Jordan Pond, the fog started to thin out a bit, giving us hope for a better view from atop Cadillac Mountain.

The elevation at Cadillac Mountain was 1,530 feet, the highest point along the North Atlantic seaboard, and the first place the sun rises in the U.S. during the fall and winter months.

Because we had a l o n g drive ahead to Montreal, we had to cut short our sightseeing at Acadia. But we couldn't leave Maine without one more taste of lobster, and some roadside wild blueberries for the trip up north.

Montreal 8-16-16

The drive from Maine to Montreal was long, but scenic. It was overcast and rainy much of the time, but that didn't dampen our spirits. For quite some time as we got close to the Canadian border, we drove alongside the Kennebec River, the most popular in Maine for whitewater rafting.

Crossing the border was easy. I didn't know what to expect, as I've never driven into another country before. The border agents checked our passports, asked what the purpose of our travel was, and sent us on our way… with a smile.

Finding our way around the province of Quebec was a little more challenging, even with navigation, as all the road signs were in French. Thank you Google Translate!

As we approached Old Montreal, the traffic specialist in me couldn't help but notice the reversible rush hour lane on the Jacque Cartier Bridge; similar to our Kennedy Expressway!

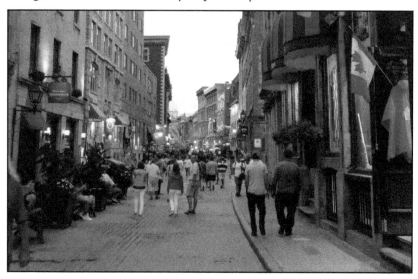

Old Montréal is the oldest area of the city. On the banks of the St. Lawrence River, it was founded in 642 by French settlers. We barely had time to explore the quaint shops along Rue St. Paul and take in the charm of Vieux Montréal.

Our dinner—c'est magnifique! Delicious steak and French wine at Vieux-Port Steakhouse was just what we needed after a long day of travel. By the way, best créme brûlée I've ever had. Our server, Steve Bellows, was delightful and gave us helpful tips on our upcoming Canadian travels. Merci beaucoup.

Toronto 8-16-16

Clear skies greeted us as we prepared to make our way Toronto. Luckily for me, Old Montréal had a modern Starbucks around the corner from our hotel. Once I was fully caffeinated, we hit the road for another long drive. We knew immediately when we crossed into Ontario, as the street signs were primarily in English.

The front end of our six-hour drive reminded me of the Midwest—flat land, lots of open space and farms. Yes, we passed construction, no it didn't cause nearly the delays we see in Chicago. Millennials didn't say "Are we there yet?" Instead, they cracked wise on Instagram.

As we approached the city, the skies became overcast, but the skyline was still visible, giving it a very urban feel.

Our hotel was within walking distance of everything we wanted to do in Toronto—shop and eat! The city reminded me very much of Chicago—crowded, but not too, bright and busy with an energetic vibe. A nice cross between Chicago and New York.

We did some power shopping at Eaton Centre, an urban mall with over 300 stores and restaurants. It attracts about a million visitors each week.

Across the street from the mall was the juxtaposition of historic and modern; the majestic Old City Hall built in 1899 in the Romanesque Revival style next to Toronto's version of Divvy bikes.

We let Sara choose our dinner destination—she picked a winner. Not only was the food terrific at The Keg Steakhouse + Bar, but the mansion also had great Canadian history.

The Keg Mansion was built in 1867, and in 1882, become home to one of Canada's most illustrious families, the Massey's. It was our delightful and animated server, Vanessa, who clued us in that the mansion was haunted. Hart Massey's daughter Lillian passed away in her bedroom, which is now the women's washroom. Her presence is said to be felt through toilets that spontaneously flush, flickering lights and the feeling of a cool breeze.

I waited until we returned to our hotel to use the facilities…just sayin'!

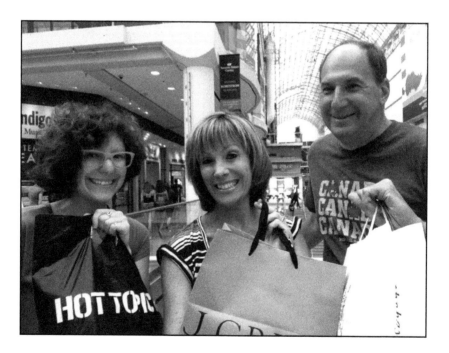

Niagara Falls 8-16-16

It was another rainy start to the day as we pulled out of Toronto, heading toward our final destination, Niagara Falls. We drove along Lake Ontario to grab a few pics, including the CN Tower, which was still visible through the mist.

As we entered the Queen Elizabeth Way (QEW) to Niagara, the rain stopped and the sun broke through, giving us incentive to make a quick stop in the city of St. Catharines to do a tasting at one of the many wineries in the region.

The wine at Chateau Des Charmes was SO tasty, we ended up buying a couple bottles.

Since we had gotten off the highway, we decided to take the back roads for the remaining nine miles or so to our hotel—good decision, GREAT scenery.

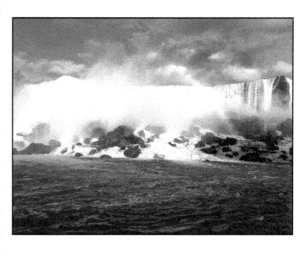

The view from our hotel room was breathtaking!

We immediately got on a tour to see the Falls up close and personal, along with a soaking boat ride. Words cannot describe the magnificence of this natural wonder.

Located on the Niagara River, which drains Lake Erie into Lake Ontario, Niagara Falls contains the largest volume (20%) of the world's fresh water. The American Falls are 880 feet across, the Canadian

(Horseshoe) Falls are 2,200 feet across. The water at both falls combined falls at a rate of 100,000 gallons PER SECOND!

There is no shortage of beauty in this region of the world.

Zip Lining along Niagara Falls
8-17-16

Nothing like going out with a bang. The "WildPlay MistRider Zipline To The Falls" had just opened and we were fortunate enough to be in the right place at the right time to give it a try. First, we made our way through Niagara Parks, a beautiful area unto its own across from the falls.

The downtown area of Niagara had a very touristy feel to it—reminding me a lot of our own Wisconsin Dells. We rode the Niagara Sky Wheel—at 175 feet, this 10-minute ride gave us another spectacular view of the falls and downtown Niagara.

As we made our way to the Zipline kiosk, my nerves were just a tad unsettled. I had been zip lining before, but this was quite different. Some 220 feet above the Niagara Gorge, riders are actually seated in a custom made harness as they zip 2,200 feet at 40 mph in roughly one minute. It turned out to be an amazing experience—not frightening, but exhilarating! I felt like I was floating alongside of one of nature's masterpieces.

Much thanks to Lindsay Di Cosimo at WildPlay Niagara Falls for setting this up, and allowing us to capture several points of view.

It was still early enough in the day to catch one more sight—we opted for the White Water Walk along the Niagara River to see the powerful rapids.

Surrounded by 410-million year old rock layers, the water rushed by at speeds of approximately 24 mph to 67 mph creating Class 6 (the most dangerous) whitewater rapids.

The distinct green color of the water is due to erosion—an estimated 60 tons of dissolved minerals are swept over Niagara Falls every minute. The green hue comes from the dissolved salts and finely ground rock from the limestone bed, shales, and sandstones.

I don't think we could have packed any more into one day. We took the Falls Incline Railway—a nice little shortcut—back to our hotel.

It was a late dinner at Canyon Creek Chophouse, and we were trying to time it so we could see the Fireworks over the Falls at 10:00 p.m. Kudos to our server Ryan, for 1) recommending the Chipotle Sirloin and 2) showing us the super-secret spot for perfect fireworks viewing. And he's a Bulls fan!

Since we had to walk past the casino to get back to our hotel, and the legal age for gambling in Canada was 19, what the heck...Sara and I played the penny slots just for kicks!

Twelve days, seven states, three Canadian cities and 2,200 miles later our road trip came to an end. One last sunrise over Niagara before we headed home to Chicago.

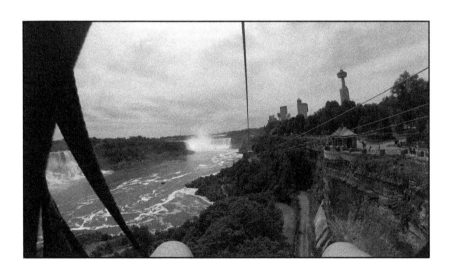

Life

The Circle of Life 1-22-17

Speaking on behalf of pet owners everywhere, I can say with confidence the tremendous joy and unconditional love we receive from our fur babies is worth the heartbreak we feel when they cross the Rainbow Bridge. I recently experienced the emotional rollercoaster of losing a cherished pet.

I had been the pet-parent to two Whippets, 13-year-old Gracie and 8-year-old Ella.

They had been in our home since they were puppies, and we looked forward to more than a dozen years apiece of love and companionship.

Gracie was the Alpha-Dog when we got Ella, but that soon changed. We affectionately called Ella "Demon Dog" because of all the mischief she got into. That dog had personality-plus!

It didn't take long for Gracie and Ella to become thick as thieves. They did everything together, went everywhere together. If one had to go to the vet, we brought the other one with for moral support. (Whippets in general suffer from separation anxiety.)

In August of 2016, shortly before Gracie's 13th birthday, we got a terrible scare. We'd been monitoring a slight heart murmur for years, but seemingly out of nowhere it worsened. Gracie was having such trouble breathing we thought she wasn't going to make it.

When I posted this on social media, I was overwhelmed with the number of people recommending that we take her to see Veterinary Cardiologist Dr. Michael Luethy at MedVet in Chicago. We rushed her to their ER the next morning. Dr. Luethy thoroughly explained her heart condition and the medications he was prescribing to treat it. Thankfully, Gracie responded incredibly well to the meds and was acting like a healthy senior dog.

Even though Gracie was on the mend, in my mind I had to prepare for the inevitable. She turned 13 in November and the life span of a healthy Whippet is about 14 or 15. I promised myself I would keep things going as long as she had a good quality of life. I was totally unprepared for what was about to happen a couple months down the road.

We noticed Ella making odd sneezing sounds; her left eye seemed to be "lazy" and not quite straight. We eventually took her to Veterinary Specialty Center in Buffalo Grove for a CT to see what was going on. The results were so catastrophic it was mind numbing.

Ella had a cancerous nasal tumor that had spread behind her eye, into her brain and through the bony tissue in her jaw. It was so large, it was inoperable. All we could do was give her pain medication until it was time. We were devastated. She was only eight. I cried until I thought there were no tears left. I was wrong. In just two weeks we had to make the difficult decision. I would not let my precious girl suffer. On January 19, 2017, Ella crossed the Rainbow Bridge.

We were heartbroken, but our Gracie was lost. Here I had been preparing for Gracie's condition to worsen. Instead, I was desperately trying to comfort her after she lost her buddy. There was only one thing to do. Find a new companion. We were fortunate that Ella's first owner had a three-year-old female Whippet named Sassi she was willing to part with to ease all of our broken hearts.

This little brindle bundle of joy was so sweet, so loving and so respectful of Gracie, who once again had become the Alpha Dog.

We will always love Ella; I feel her presence throughout my home. Her spirit is with me when I walk Gracie, as if to say, "Don't worry Mom, you

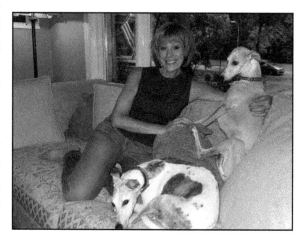

gave me a great life, I'm no longer in pain, it's going to be okay. Take care of Sassi now." (Sassi's father is Ella's half-brother.)

And such is The Circle Of Life.

Epilogue

We have always been a two-dog family. It was difficult enough losing Ella to cancer when she was only eight years old, but then to lose our other dog, Gracie, less than four months later, was nearly unbearable.

That's why it's taken me a little longer to write about Gracie. The grieving process was rougher because she was the first dog I owned as an adult. I'll never forget when we discovered her in a room full of puppies. Gracie ran to me and wouldn't stop licking my face. I would always tell people, "I didn't choose her—she chose me!"

After Glenn and I married in 2005, it didn't take long for Gracie to fit right into our blended family. Gracie bonded with Zelda (Glenn's Airedale) as Sara bonded with Colin and Tyler (Glenn's sons).

Unfortunately, just a few short years later, we lost Zelda to cancer. Gracie was inconsolable. It broke my heart, seeing her stand by the car, waiting for her buddy to jump out. We *had* to get another dog. One month later, we welcomed Ella, our second Whippet.

Ella gave Gracie a run for her money, not doubt. Gracie eventually gave in to the power struggle, but the two became fast and furious friends, never wanting to be separated.

Gracie was an incredibly smart and loving dog, but she also had her unique traits. This dog was the definition of anxiety! We couldn't crate-train her. Every car ride was filled with her panting and drooling, and don't even get me started on thunderstorms. (Yes we tried the ThunderShirt. No it didn't work.)

Gracie was definitely my dog, and very tolerant of being in the spotlight. She and Ella accompanied me to many Anti-Cruelty Society Bark In The Park fundraisers. She was a Bears fan when we hoped they'd win, and a Cubs fan when they finally did!

Gracie loved spending time at our place in Wisconsin (once she got past that long car ride up there) to join me in the peddle boat, or sun-bathe on the deck. The heat was never too much for her.

In her younger days she chased (and caught) squirrels and chip-munks. She co-starred in a dog show pilot that never aired, and was front and center in a fundraiser photo shoot that did make it to print.

In her later years she was by my side, providing comfort as only a canine companion can.

By Gracie's 13th birthday, an ongoing heart condition was being kept under control with medication. I started to prepare myself for the inevi-table. Instead, I was dealt the unimaginable when my younger dog Ella was diagnosed with, and soon after, passed away from cancer.

We were lucky enough to bring three-year old Sassi into our home as a companion for Gracie in her final months. As Gracie's condition worsened, I had to make to the decision. I couldn't believe I was doing this again, so soon. Saying goodbye was more painful than I could have ever imagined.

My heart was heavy, but Sassi was there to help it heal. We immedi-ately started the search for a new puppy to fill the void. Enter Lola! We flew to North Carolina to get this four-month-old Whippet pup, and then drove back home to Chicago in one weekend.

As the puppy training and canine bonding process began again, we have taken on our roles as fur parents with renewed vigor and the same uncon-ditional love our fur babies have given to us.

I wouldn't have it any other way.

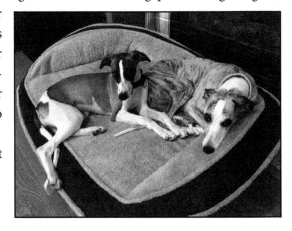

About the Author

Traffic/Transportation Anchor Roz Varon was the first in the country to bring traffic rush hour reporting to TV morning news. She joined ABC 7 News as Morning Traffic Anchor in April 1989. Roz not only updates Chicagoans on snarls and travel times, but she also provides extensive coverage of the transportation beat.

Roz has won multiple Emmy Awards in Traffic Reporting, Specialty Programming, Spot News and Features. Also, she was honored with a Peter Lisagor Award for her "Weekender" series, a weekly roundup of metro Chicago events. The Girl Scouts recognized her as a role model with their "Girls Scouts of the USA Thanks Badge." Additionally, she won the Illinois Broadcasters Association's Silver Dome Award for her breast cancer special, "Faces of Inspiration."

As a breast cancer survivor, Roz works diligently to help heighten cancer prevention and awareness and is an in-demand motivational speaker. An animal lover, she volunteers much of her time to the Anti-Cruelty Society and PAWS Chicago.

Since 2000, Roz has served on the Board of Governors of the Chicago/Midwest Chapter of the National Academy of Television Arts & Sciences.

She received a B.A. in Broadcast Communications from Columbia College, and resides in the western suburbs of Chicago with her husband, daughter, two dogs and a cat.